# THE LUPUS DIET PLAN

Shrimp Scampi on Zucchini Noodles, p. 154

# The LUPUS Diet Plan

Meal Plans & Recipes to
Soothe Inflammation, Treat Flares,
and Send Lupus into Remission

*Laura Rellihan, RD*

ROCKRIDGE
PRESS

*I dedicate this book to my mother,*
*my father, and my husband Patrick,*
*who all stood by me through my*
*hardest days and always encouraged me*
*to keep pursuing my dreams.*

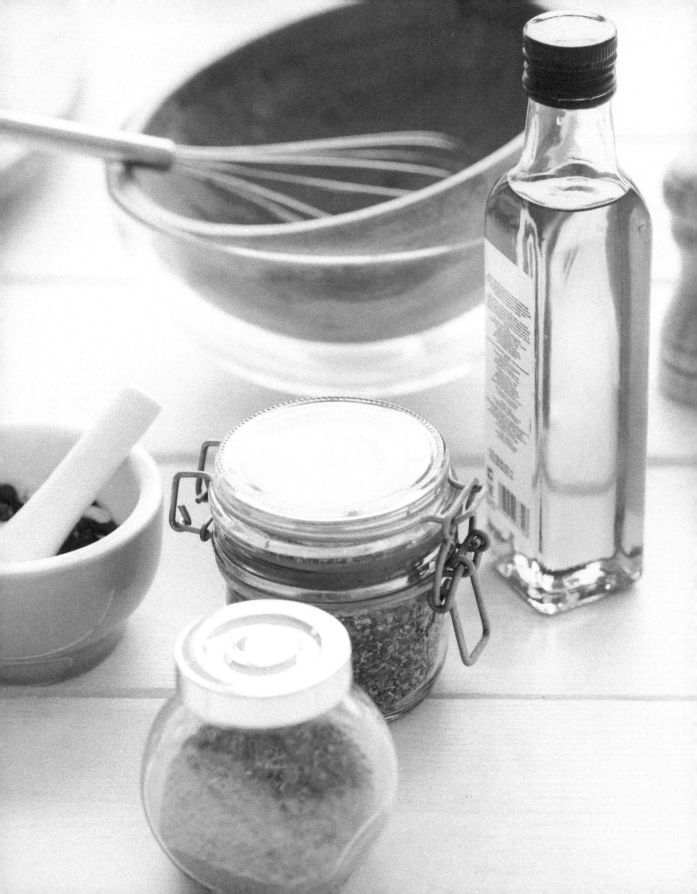

# Contents

# Foreword

Whether you are newly diagnosed with lupus or you have had the disease for decades, *The Lupus Diet Plan* is a must-have addition to your cooking and lifestyle book collection.

Living with systemic lupus for 26 years, I have been through it all. Throughout the duration of my illness, I have been hospitalized dozens of times, had many surgeries for joint and kidney issues, and have suffered from painful lung conditions. I know firsthand how hard the daily struggle of life with lupus can be. I also know that the foods I eat can directly impact my levels of inflammation, pain, and fatigue.

Sadly, I lived many of my early years with lupus not understanding the connection between the food I ate and the inflammation affecting my health. I took pill after pill in hopes of finding relief from the devastating symptoms of my illness. If I had been given something like this book earlier in my diagnosis, I might have been able to avoid some of the awful side effects of the many medications I was given. Don't get me wrong, I believe in Western medicine and its importance. But I also believe that the medical care we receive should work in conjunction with how we live

and what we eat and drink. All of these factors affect our health, so it's important to achieve a good balance.

In this book, Laura provides an excellent narrative that outlines easy ways to establish healthy eating habits and lifestyle choices while explaining the science behind the food. With a concise look at what lupus is, what it does, and how it affects the immune system, she guides you through the illness without overwhelming you with too much clinical medical jargon. Her medication breakdown is exceptionally helpful for those who are newly diagnosed, and I love that she includes a worksheet for practicing gratitude daily.

Rather than focusing on the foods we can't have, she focuses on all the delectable foods we can eat, by providing us with simple, colorful, and mouthwatering recipes. Many of these recipes can be modified so that they're easier to prepare when we're experiencing a flare and feeling especially exhausted and uncomfortable, and they include substitution tips for readers who need to eat in a way that supports their bone health, cardiovascular health, or kidney health, too.

In an age when doctors' visits are getting shorter and shorter, we often leave our appointment not knowing what to do after receiving a lupus diagnosis. We leave feeling helpless and hopeless. It is refreshing and reassuring to know we now have a guide for answering the question, *"How can I be proactive with my own health?"* Laura gives us straightforward examples of how to be proactive through nutrition and more! And her answer is simple: what you invest in your health, you will get back. The first step in this investment is simple, too—use this book!

## ABOUT THE FOREWORD CONTRIBUTOR

KELLI ROSETA is the Client Services Coordinator for Molly's Fund Fighting Lupus, a national nonprofit dedicated to educating the public and medical community about lupus. A 26-year systemic lupus erythematosus survivor and the award-winning blog contributor for Molly's Fund Fighting Lupus, Kelli dedicates her time to supporting those living with lupus and affirming them in their journey. As the facilitator for their online Facebook support chats and in-person patient support groups, Kelli's goal is to help others feel like they are not alone and to discover joy within their "new normal."

# Introduction

Sometimes I sit back and wonder what my life would be like if I had never been diagnosed with lupus. Then I realize how far I have come, and I think that being diagnosed with lupus may have been the best thing that ever happened to me. I know what you're thinking—it's a horrible disease! But I am a glass-half-full kind of girl. Without lupus, I would never have found my passion to become a registered dietitian. So the way I look at it, lupus was the beginning of my new life. You may be wondering the same thing about your own lupus diagnosis. Well, as Benjamin Franklin once said, "An investment in knowledge always pays the best interest." I hope that the insights you are about to gain from reading this book will help you realize your own potential. Just the fact that you picked up this book puts you back in the driver's seat and will hopefully give you the confidence you need to fight this debilitating disease.

In 1995, I was diagnosed with systemic lupus erythematosus nephritis, a type of lupus that affects the kidneys. I was only 15 years old and not at all focused on taking care of myself. Then suddenly I was waking up with stiff joints, developing ulcers in my mouth, feeling weak all the time, and losing my hair—which served as my wake-up call. I had to grow up fast. I had to start paying attention to what was happening to my body.

My doctors immediately started me on one of the routine medications for lupus, an intravenous steroid called Solu-Medrol (methylprednisolone). A common side effect of this drug is weight gain, and I went from 90 pounds to 180 pounds in less than six months. You can imagine what this would do to a fifteen-year-old's self-esteem, so clinical depression was soon added to the countless other symptoms I was facing. I had also been diagnosed with stage 3 chronic kidney disease.

Unlike some, though, I was fortunate to have parents who taught me the basics of nutrition when I was young. At the time, there was not much research on the role of nutrition in treating lupus, so my own experiments began. I tried drinking barley grass juice, which I thought of as "green slime." I had to hold my nose as I downed it. Thankfully that experiment did not last long, and soon I began to learn about whole foods and the roles they play in combating disease.

I started to realize that without good nutrition, my health and quality of life would not allow me to enjoy even the simplest of daily activities. After I modified my diet on my own, my doctors and I noticed huge improvements in my lab results—and in how I felt. As a bonus, my kidney function started to improve, and slowly but surely I could start living my life again and be more active.

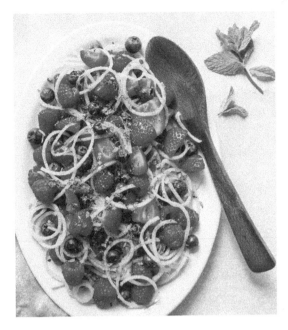 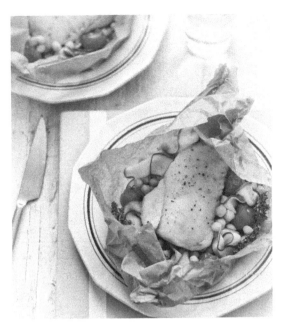

During my college years, I developed a further interest in nutrition and its effect on disease, and I eventually became a registered dietitian. My own health background provides me with a better understanding of my clients' personal struggles, and I enjoy helping them achieve success in attaining their nutrition and health goals.

For some of us, even the idea of cooking causes stress, not to mention all the slicing, dicing, and sautéing. Fortunately, it's a myth that only a chef or culinary expert can produce a delicious meal using high-quality ingredients. The recipes in this cookbook are geared toward people with lupus, who might be dealing with pain and fatigue. The dishes are affordable and easy to prepare, even for those who think there's no time for cooking in their busy lives. Also included in this book are meal plans for people with various dietary restrictions related to kidney health, bone health, and cardiovascular issues.

It's time to start looking at your own glass as half full. Fill it all the way to the top with knowledge and good nutrition, and you, too, can overcome lupus. Your body is an investment that you'll have for life, so take good care of it.

# Part One

## LEARNING TO MANAGE LUPUS

If you're holding this book in your hand, chances are that you (or someone you love) have been diagnosed with lupus.

In the chapters that follow, you'll learn about the different types of lupus and the complications they can present. You'll get a basic overview of dietary guidelines for managing symptoms, and additional nutritional guidance for complications such as organ damage or medicinal side effects. Handy food lists will teach you which ingredients to enjoy and avoid. By following a meal plan for several weeks, you'll learn to eat in a way that calms your symptoms and supports your health goals. And because nutrition is not the only factor for managing lupus, you'll learn important lifestyle tips for getting adequate rest, managing stress, and staying physically active.

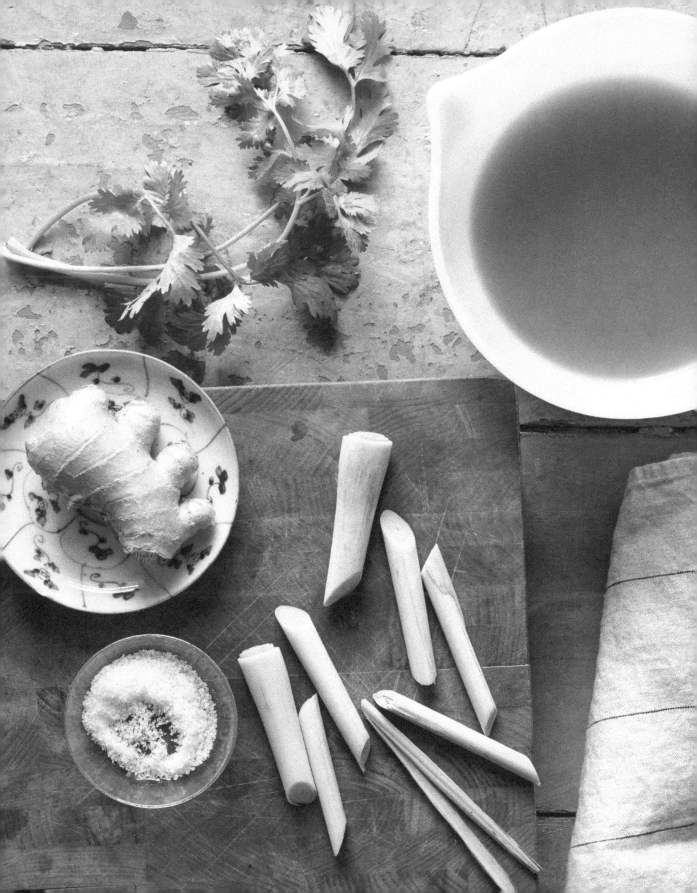

# 1

# The Lupus-Diet Connection

Lupus is an especially difficult disease to diagnose, and flares can be unpredictable. You never know how bad a flare will be or how long it will last. It can develop rapidly or slowly, and sometimes the symptoms are not even noticeable. As complicated as this disease is, you should not let lupus govern your life or your attitude.

This chapter covers the basics of the immune system, complications and symptoms associated with lupus, and coexisting conditions such as kidney damage, high blood pressure, and anemia. There's also an overview of the basics of the anti-inflammatory diet for people with lupus, along with helpful tips. Before starting any new diet or lifestyle routine, be sure to discuss it with your health care provider.

## How the Immune System Works

A healthy, normal immune system works to protect the body against harmful influences from the environment, such as germs, bacteria, parasites, and viruses. A normal immune system makes proteins called antibodies that protect the body from these intruders. If there is a problem with the immune system, diseases such as lupus can result.

Lupus is an autoimmune disease that can lead to harm in any area of the body (such as skin, joints, and internal organs). An autoimmune disease is one in which the immune system is unable to distinguish between harmful foreign invaders and the body's own tissue. The body's antibodies then attack the healthy tissue in addition to or instead of the intruders. This results in pain and chronic inflammation, which can lead to tissue or organ damage if left uncontrolled.

There are four types of lupus:

1. *Discoid lupus erythematosus* produces a chronic skin rash but does not attack other major organs of the body.

2. *Subacute cutaneous lupus erythematosus* causes skin sores on areas of the body that are exposed to the sun.

3. *Neonatal lupus* is rare and is found only in newborns of a mom with lupus. Symptoms usually cease after a few months.

4. *Systemic lupus erythematosus,* the most common form of lupus, is considered the most serious because it often affects major organs of the body, such as the kidneys, heart, brain, lungs, blood, and skin. Because of organ damage and side effects from medications, coexisting conditions can occur, such as high blood pressure, anemia, osteoporosis, weight gain, and kidney disease.

## Symptoms, Flares, and Complications

Lupus is hard to diagnose because symptoms can vary from one person to another and can change quickly. The most common symptoms include joint pain and swelling, skin rashes (especially a "butterfly" rash on the face), photosensitivity, and fatigue. Other less common symptoms include hair loss, anemia (a decrease in red blood cells), chest pain, mouth ulcers, and Raynaud's syndrome (numbness and color changes in fingers and toes from cold and stress). Some people with lupus experience headaches, seizures, depression, dizziness, and confusion.

During times of remission, these symptoms are under control, but they return during a flare-up—often with the addition of new symptoms. Although prolonged remission of lupus is rare, with additional research and new treatments, it is now possible for some. Researchers have also learned more about how diet affects people with lupus, leading to an overall improvement in their quality of life.

In this book, you will find healthy and delicious recipes specifically developed to meet your individual needs and nutrient requirements. The three unique meal plans will assist you in maintaining good health with easy and nutritious recipes to help you fight inflammation and take care of yourself during a flare.

# CONSIDERATIONS FOR THE NEWLY DIAGNOSED

Have you just been diagnosed with lupus? Maybe you are scared or confused, or maybe you are relieved to finally be able to put a name to your illness. Even though lupus is a serious disease and should be closely monitored, there is no reason you cannot live a full life. Take advantage of these five practical tips to track and manage your lupus:

1. **Find a doctor who specializes in autoimmune diseases.** Because lupus is a very complicated disease, ideally your doctor will specialize in lupus and be familiar with the current research and treatments. It is very important to establish a good relationship with your doctor and be honest about your symptoms and side effects.

2. **Do your research.** Look for up-to-date research. The Lupus Foundation of America (lupus.org) and Molly's Fund Fighting Lupus (www.mollysfund.org) are both great places to start.

3. **Reach out.** You are not alone! According to the Lupus Foundation of America, it is estimated that 1.5 million Americans and at least 5 million people worldwide have a form of lupus. Start with your local community or join a social media support group. One good resource is Molly's Fund Fighting Lupus, which runs programs for both local, in-person support groups and online support groups that use Facebook chat. It is also important to reach out to family and friends, so they can understand and help you cope with your condition.

4. **Be good to yourself.** The most important thing you can do for yourself is listen to your body. Take care of yourself by developing healthy habits such as good nutrition, proper sleep habits, and regular exercise.

5. **Manage your stress.** Stress can aggravate your lupus symptoms, so it's important to learn what causes stress in your life and what helps you cope with your stress. Consider practicing deep breathing techniques or meditation exercises.

# The Anti-Inflammatory Diet for Lupus

Since lupus is a chronic inflammatory disease, there has been growing interest in the role of nutrition and its influence on the inflammatory response. While there are no foods that are known to cause or cure lupus, research shows that a diet high in vitamins, minerals, and monounsaturated and polyunsaturated fatty acids can have beneficial effects against tissue damage and inflammatory activity. Diet therapy can offer people with lupus a better quality of life and can also help treat or prevent other coexisting conditions such as high blood pressure, osteoporosis, cardiac disease, and chronic kidney disease.

## DIETARY GUIDELINES FOR MANAGING LUPUS

- *Balance your nutrients.* Each meal should include at least 2 to 3 ounces of quality protein (eggs, fish, legumes/beans, lean meats, and nuts/seeds), one serving of vegetable or fruits from the approved list, and one serving of the approved carbohydrates.

- *Monitor your calories and manage your weight.* Excessive weight gain in lupus patients who are on chronic steroids has been found to contribute to high blood pressure, further joint stress, cardiovascular disease, and other conditions.

- *Increase your intake of fruits and vegetables.* See the table on pages 22 to 23. You may want to consider limiting nightshade vegetables because they can negatively affect some people with lupus. The main nightshades to avoid are white potatoes, sweet and hot peppers, tomatoes, tomatillos, and eggplant.

- *Switch to healthy fats.* Omega-3 and omega-6 fatty acids contain anti-inflammatory properties and can also help raise "good" cholesterol (HDL) to help prevent heart disease. Good sources of these unsaturated fatty acids include fatty fish, fish oil supplements, walnuts and walnut oil, canola oil, flaxseed meal and flaxseed oil, and avocados.

- *Focus on fiber.* Fiber helps lower cholesterol and lipid levels and protect against cardiovascular disease. Fiber also helps increase absorption of minerals such as calcium. The daily recommendation for fiber is 25 to 30 grams per day. Good fiber sources are fruits, vegetables, whole grains, nuts, and seeds.

- *Choose whole grains.* Whole grains are a good source of fiber, energy, and B vitamins, and are also low in fat. Whole-grain foods include whole-wheat bread and pasta, rye, oats, and barley. If you have celiac or gluten intolerance, there are plenty of gluten-free whole grains, such as amaranth, brown rice, wild rice, farro, and buckwheat.

- *Stay hydrated.* Our bodies are composed of 70 percent water, and we need to constantly replenish it. It is recommended that you drink at least eight cups of water per day. Add two more cups of water on days that you are exercising or sweating profusely. If you suffer from kidney or cardiac issues, check with your health care provider, as these conditions may impair your excretion of water and require you to limit your fluid intake.

- *Watch your caffeine intake.* Although black and green teas can provide anti-inflammatory benefits, caffeine can decrease your iron absorption. Since anemia is a common issue with people who have lupus, it's important to limit your caffeine intake.

## EATING FOR COMPLICATIONS OR COEXISTING CONDITIONS

Many lupus patients suffer from coexisting conditions, and they may need to make further changes to their diet. Chapter 3 features three unique meal plans that will help reduce complications from coexisting conditions such as lupus-related kidney disease, as well as assist you through a lupus flare. In addition, every recipe in this book is gluten-free.

- *Basic Lupus Diet Meal Plan:* General anti-inflammatory diet recipes for people with lupus who want to maintain good health.

- *Flare & Fatigue Meal Plan:* Easy anti-inflammatory recipes to minimize fatigue and pain; the recipes are also free of potentially aggravating ingredients such as gluten, the big 8 allergens, and nightshades.

- *Kidney Support Meal Plan:* Recipes that are not only anti-inflammatory but are also low in sodium and phosphorus to help manage kidney disease.

The following sections discuss which nutrients help maintain good health, and which foods are the best sources of these nutrients. To help you remember this information, turn to The Lupus Diet Food Lists on pages 22 to 23. Keep this table on hand as a reference when you go grocery shopping.

## FOODS THAT NOURISH AND HEAL

- *Vitamin A* contains anti-inflammatory properties. Food sources: sweet potatoes, carrots, winter squashes, romaine lettuce, dark leafy greens, bell peppers, dried apricots, tropical fruits, cantaloupe, fish, and liver.

- *Vitamin D* levels may be low in people with lupus because their photosensitivity causes them to avoid direct sunlight, which is the main source of this important nutrient. Low levels of vitamin D are related to inflammatory activity in lupus, whereas high levels have been associated with reduction of symptoms. Food sources: fortified milk, egg yolks, salmon, tuna, sardines, and herring.

- *Vitamin E* delays the appearance of auto-immunity and increases survival. Food sources: whole grains, nuts, raw seeds, dark leafy greens, broccoli, avocados, squash, pumpkin, fruit, shellfish, and fish.

- *Vitamin C* helps decrease the risk of cardiovascular disease, inflammation, and oxidative stress, which can cause tissue and organ damage. Food sources: citrus fruits, strawberries, cantaloupe, tomatoes, bell peppers, broccoli, cauliflower, and cabbage.

# Medication: Side Effects and Dietary Advice

| MEDICATION | POSSIBLE SIDE EFFECTS | DIETARY ADVICE |
|---|---|---|
| **Corticosteroids** (prednisone, methylprednisolone, cortisone, hydrocortisone) | Increased appetite; fluid retention; weight gain; bone mineral depletion; high blood pressure; problems with mood, memory, and behavior; other psychological effects | Consume calcium-fortified foods or take a supplement. Consume nutrient-dense, low-calorie foods such as fruits and vegetables. Manage weight through diet and exercise. Follow a low-sodium diet (2,000 mg/day). |
| **Diuretics** | Low sodium in the blood (hyponatremia), dizziness, headaches, dehydration, electrolyte imbalance, muscle cramps, gout and other joint disorders, impotence | Stay hydrated. Avoid salty foods. Manage weight through diet and exercise. Avoid alcohol. For gout, follow a low-purine diet (limit meat and seafood to about 3 ounces per meal). |
| **Nonsteroidal anti-inflammatory drugs** (NSAIDs) (ibuprofen, aspirin, naproxen) | Stomach irritation, GI ulcers | Consume probiotics or fermented foods. Take medicine with food or antacid to avoid stomach upset. |
| **Anti-malarial drugs** | Retinol toxicity | N/A |
| **Immunosuppressive drugs** (methotrexate, azathioprine, cyclophosphamide) | Nausea, indigestion, mouth sores, hair loss | Avoid alcohol. Eat a balanced diet full of vitamins, minerals, and antioxidants. |
| **Anticoagulants** (aspirin, warfarin, and other blood thinners) | Indigestion, diarrhea, constipation, hair loss | Avoid alcohol. Consume adequate fiber (25–30 g/day). Consume probiotics or fermented foods. |

- *Calcium* intake is especially important for lupus patients who are taking corticosteroids, which interfere with the absorption of calcium and can lead to osteoporosis. Food sources: milk, broccoli, cabbage, sauerkraut, dark leafy greens, rutabaga, legumes, tofu, and salmon.

- *Omega-3 and omega-6 fatty acids,* also known as eicosapentaenoic acid (EPA) and docosahexaenoic acid (DHA), produce an enzyme called lipoxygenase that aids in the reduction of the inflammatory process. Studies have also shown that they help protect against cardiovascular problems. Food sources: salmon, mackerel, sardines, herring, flaxseed oil, avocados, nuts, and seeds.

- *Green and black teas* have anti-inflammatory properties and help balance hormone levels, which can fend off stress. However, if you have anemia, it's important to limit consumption of caffeinated products or drink only decaffeinated tea.

- *Probiotics* are the beneficial bacteria in the gut. Research suggests a potential link between consumption of the *Lactobacillus* bacteria, found primarily in yogurt cultures, and a decrease in lupus activity. Food sources: yogurt and fermented foods.

## FOODS THAT TRIGGER AND INFLAME

- *Processed foods* tend to be high in salt, sugar, and refined and simple carbohydrates. These types of carbohydrates can often worsen the side effects of some medications and contribute to poor blood glucose control and fatigue. In addition, when food is processed, valuable nutrients such as fiber and vitamins are often removed. Your best bet is to eat fresh, whole foods whenever possible.

- *Excessive protein* can be problematic if you have lupus-related kidney disease. While a moderate amount of protein is essential to a healthy diet, research shows that a diet too high in protein can contribute to further kidney damage.

- *Sodium* intake needs to be cut back, especially if you have high blood pressure or kidney disease. And if you are taking corticosteroids, a low-sodium diet will help you combat the fluid retention common with these medications.

- *Saturated fats* should be reduced. High levels of saturated fat in the blood coupled with an increase in inflammation-induced tissue damage can lead to cardiovascular disease.

- *Trans fats* raise "bad" cholesterol (LDL) levels and can increase the risk of cardiovascular disease. Trans fats are found mostly in commercial baked goods such as crackers, cookies, cakes, doughnuts, muffins, and pies. Avoid products with "partially hydrogenated" oils in their list of ingredients.

- *Alfalfa* is high in L-canavanine, which research suggests can increase antibody production and reactivate clinical symptoms related to lupus. Alfalfa sprouts are sometimes used as a topping on salads or sandwiches at delis and cafés.

# The Lupus Diet Food Lists

| FOOD GROUP | ENJOY FREELY | LIMIT | AVOID |
|---|---|---|---|
| **Allium vegetables** | chives, *onions, scallions, shallots | fresh garlic | supplemental garlic |
| **Cruciferous vegetables** | *broccoli, Brussels sprouts, *cabbage *cauliflower, kale | | frozen vegetables with high-sodium sauces or seasonings |
| **Dark, leafy greens** | *arugula, collard greens, *kale, lettuces, mustard greens, romaine, *spinach, Swiss chard | | alfalfa, frozen vegetables with high-sodium sauces or seasonings |
| **Nightshade vegetables** | | eggplant, sweet or hot peppers, tomatillos, tomatoes, white potatoes | |
| **Root vegetables** | *beets, carrots, celery root, kohlrabi, parsnips, rutabaga, *sweet potatoes, turnips, *yams | | frozen vegetables with high-sodium sauces or seasonings |
| **Winter squashes** | acorn, *butternut, delicata, hubbard, kabocha, *pumpkin, spaghetti squash | | |
| **Fruit** | apples, banana, blackberries, *blueberries, cherries, clementines, grapefruit, kiwi, lemon, mango, nectarines, oranges, peaches, pineapple, strawberries, tangerines | canned fruit in juice | canned fruit with added syrup |
| **Beans and legumes** | choose dried or low-sodium/no-salt-added canned beans: adzuki, *black, kidney, lentils, lima, navy, split peas | chickpeas, fava beans, kudzu, soy | canned beans with added salt or high-sodium seasonings |

# The Lupus Diet Food Lists

| FOOD GROUP | ENJOY FREELY | LIMIT | AVOID |
|---|---|---|---|
| **Grains** | amaranth, arrowroot, barley, *brown rice, *buckwheat, bulgur, corn, cornmeal, couscous, farina, farro, flax, gluten-free flours (rice, soy, corn, potato, bean), kamut, millet, *quinoa, semolina, sorghum, spelt, tapioca, teff, triticale, wheat, wild rice | | If following gluten-free diet, avoid barley, malt, malt flavoring, malt vinegar, bulgur, durum flour, graham flour, couscous, farina, farro, kamut, oats, rye, semolina, spelt, triticale, and wheat |
| **Animal products** | beef (grass-fed), chicken, eggs, halibut, lamb, mackerel, pork (lean), *salmon, sardines, trout, tuna, turkey, yogurt | butter, cheese, cream, ice cream, milk | cured meats/fish high in salt (bacon, salami, anchovies, smoked salmon) |
| **Nuts and seeds** | almonds, Brazil nuts, cashews, *chia seeds, *flaxseed, *hemp seeds, macadamia nuts, pumpkin seeds, sesame seeds, *walnuts | peanuts | salted or artificially flavored nuts and seeds |
| **Fats and oils** | avocado and avocado oil, *coconut oil, *extra-virgin olive oil, *flaxseed oil, ghee (if tolerated), hemp oil | margarine and corn, peanut, canola, soybean, and vegetable oils | |
| **Herbs and spices** | *basil, cilantro, *cinnamon, *cloves, cumin, dill, fennel seeds, *ginger, nutmeg, oregano, parsley, rosemary, sage, thyme, *turmeric | | herb and spice blends with added salt |
| **Sweeteners** | coconut sugar, honey, maple syrup (pure), molasses, stevia | brown sugar, corn syrup, granulated sugar | artificial sweeteners (Splenda/sucralose, Nutra-Sweet/aspartame, sorbitol, xylitol, maltodextrin) |

*Foods marked with an asterisk are particularly powerful at fighting inflammation.

- **Alcohol** can lower the effectiveness of some medications, cause additional health problems, and worsen existing symptoms.

- **Caffeine** can reduce the amount of iron your body absorbs by half. Iron is important in preventing anemia, which is a common complication of lupus.

## FOODS TO CONSIDER WITH CARE

If you are unsure about how certain foods will affect you, keep a food diary and monitor your symptoms. Be sure to follow up with a dietitian or doctor before eliminating essential foods from your diet.

- **Nightshade vegetables** include white potatoes, sweet and hot peppers, tomatoes, tomatillos, and eggplant. While there is no supporting data that nightshades cause lupus flares, some people with lupus find that it helps to remove or limit these vegetables from their diet.

- **Sugar and high fructose corn syrup** in excessive amounts contributes to obesity, which can lead to metabolic complications such as diabetes and cardiovascular disease. It is also thought that sugar may trigger an inflammatory response in the body and reduce energy levels.

- **Gluten** sensitivity or celiac disease can be determined by your physician through serological testing. Regardless, if you find that avoiding gluten helps alleviate your lupus symptoms, then it makes sense to continue doing so. Most large grocery store chains now carry a wide variety of gluten-free breads, crackers, pastas, and cereals.

- **Isoflavones** are compounds found in soy, peanuts, chickpeas, fava beans, alfalfa, and kudzu. There is mixed research regarding the effects of isoflavones on lupus-related kidney damage, so consider carefully whether to consume foods containing these compounds.

- **Garlic** may stimulate the immune system, especially when taken in high-dose supplemental form. While there are no specific studies related to garlic, some people with lupus might want to avoid it in order to suppress the disease.

- **The big eight allergens**—wheat, eggs, fish, shellfish, soy, tree nuts, peanuts, and dairy—account for about 90 percent of food allergies. These foods should be eliminated from your diet only when following the recommendations of a health professional and after appropriate food allergy testing.

# Setting Reasonable Expectations

Starting a new diet regimen can be overwhelming at first, especially when making major changes to your lifestyle and diet. Remember that the meal plans in chapter 3 have done the hard work of planning for you!

## TIPS TO HELP YOU GET STARTED

- **Clean and restock your pantry.** Use the Lupus Diet Food Lists and the meal plans in chapter 3 as guides when restocking your cupboards and refrigerator to fit your new lifestyle.

- **Set reasonable goals and take it one step at a time.** For example, if you are used to eating a lot of processed foods and foods high in saturated fats, start by replacing just one processed food with a healthy snack from the approved food lists or recipes.

- **Distract yourself from cravings.** Food cravings will occur, especially if you are on corticosteroids. If you can, go for a walk or change your environment to avoid temptation. Consider drinking a glass of water to minimize the craving.

- **Remember that every day is a new day.** There will still be parties, holidays, and vacations with loads of foods you need to avoid. Plan for these events by eating beforehand or by packing a snack or meal so you can stay on track with your new lifestyle. If you happen to slip up or "cheat," try not beat yourself up about it. You can always start fresh the next day.

By making healthy choices and supporting your health, you can expect to see some wonderful long-term changes. Here are a few to look forward to:

- **Weight loss.** While weight loss depends largely on calorie intake and energy use, the lupus diet contains good sources of fiber and nutrients that will help you achieve a healthy weight. Consider speaking with a health professional to identify your specific calorie and protein requirements to help you determine your weight loss goals.

- **Increased energy levels.** Even though factors such as environment and stress may be out of your control at times, following the lupus diet will provide you with more energy.

- **Remission.** Good nutrition can result in an anti-inflammatory state, which can make it possible for remission to occur. Of course, this also depends on managing stress levels, which will be covered in chapter 2.

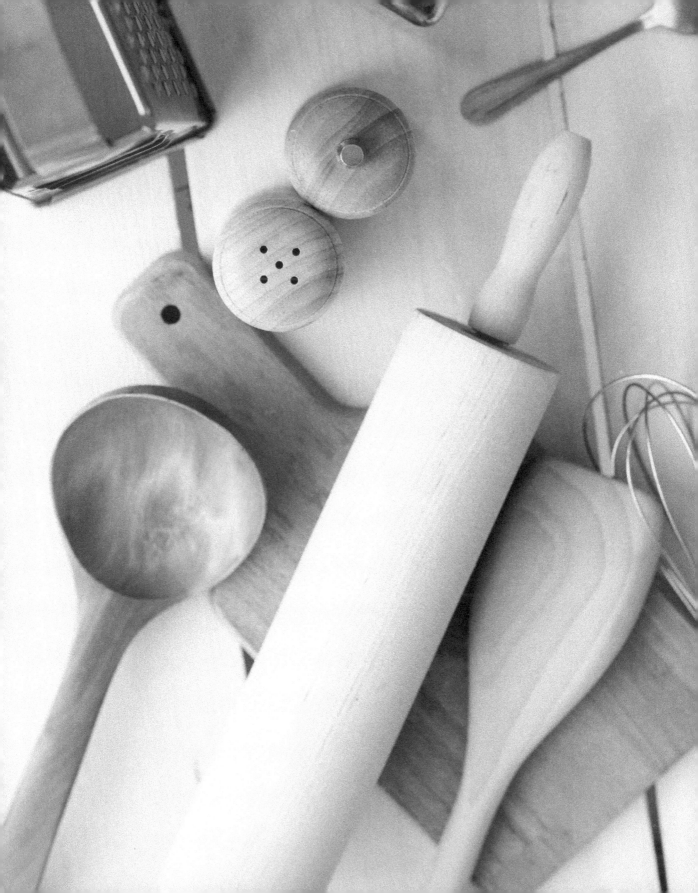

# 2

# Living Well to Eat Well

I can vividly remember walking down my high school hallway, feeling ashamed about my disease and embarrassed about who I was. You may be suffering with similar thoughts. Because of negative emotions, pain, fatigue, and stress, you may find it hard to stay motivated. If it's not depression or shame or fear, it might be joint pain and stiffness that make getting out of bed each morning a struggle. In addition to physical symptoms, lupus can affect memory and concentration, resulting in what is referred to as "lupus fog." Dealing on a day-to-day basis with these difficult conditions can discourage us from living life fully. It's true that the stresses of life will always be present, but we can learn to manage stress through healthy lifestyle habits like rest and exercise. Managing stress is critical to avoiding or minimizing a lupus flare and improving our overall quality of life.

# The Importance of a Healthy Lifestyle

Research shows that chronic psychological stress can cause the body to lose its ability to regulate the inflammatory response. That's why it is especially important for people with lupus to manage their stress levels and to start making healthy lifestyle choices in addition to dietary changes. It might seem impossible to balance sleep, exercise, and leisure time with work and family obligations, all while dealing with a chronic illness. However, the rewards of adopting healthy habits can be life changing. Imagine waking up with joy again, eager to start your day! This is entirely possible, but you will need to start listening to your body.

## REST AND SLEEP

Getting adequate rest and sleep is just as important for managing lupus as eating well and exercising. Unfortunately, according to the National Institutes of Health, some 70 million people in the United States are affected by chronic sleep disorders or intermittent sleep problems. You might be a type A personality (like me) and struggle with allowing yourself to rest. When my first child was born, I thought I could keep up with the laundry, cook dinner every night, and still compete in triathlons while getting up three times during the night to feed a newborn. By the time my second kid was born, I had started listening to my body and learned some simple methods to help me relax and rest. Proper sleep can improve your physical and mental health, as well as your body's ability to conserve energy and other resources that the immune system needs to stay strong.

Here are some simple tips to help you improve your rest and sleep habits:

- *Set a schedule.* As much as possible, try to go to bed and wake up at the same time every day. A consistent schedule will help control your body's internal clock so you can fall asleep more easily—and stay asleep.

- *Practice a relaxing routine before bed.* Our bodies crave routine. For example, if you like to take a warm bath before bed or read each night as part of your routine, this will help your body know when it is time for sleep.

- *Exercise early.* Some studies suggest that vigorous exercise too close to bedtime can elevate your heart rate and adrenaline, increasing the time it takes you to get to sleep. If you have trouble relaxing before bed and getting to sleep, then do any vigorous exercise at least two hours before your bedtime. The important thing is to find an exercise routine that relaxes you and then stick to it.

- *Avoid caffeine, alcohol, and nicotine.* Caffeine, alcohol, and nicotine work as stimulants, which make it difficult to fall asleep and stay asleep, so it's best to avoid them altogether but especially right before bed.

- *Avoid eating big meals or spicy foods late at night.* This may lead to indigestion and discomfort, which can disrupt sleep. If you are hungry, try eating a small snack at least one hour before bedtime.

# THE POWER OF HEALTHY HABITS

**If you continue to let a bad habit grow, it becomes a part of who you are. It can take 30 to 90 days to break a habit, but it's the most rewarding accomplishment!**

To break a habit, it is important to know what triggers it. Charles Duhigg, a journalist who's authored books on habits and productivity, says that the trouble with breaking a habit "is not a lack of determination—it's a lack of understanding how habit works." That is, it's important to understand what triggers the habit and why it is occurring. Then you can start replacing your harmful habits with healthy habits, which can help you on your journey with lupus, even during the most difficult times. It's never too late to adopt healthy habits! If you are having trouble breaking your bad habits and adopting good ones, try using the Gratitude and Habit Trackers on pages 30 and 31 or making your own in a journal.

Here are a few tips for changing bad habits into good ones:

1. **Identify the triggers for your habits.** For example, if you have a habit of checking Facebook at work, take a week to track what you're usually doing before you open that Facebook page. What seems to be the cue that causes you to log on?

2. **Identify the rewards that you feel when you engage in a habit.** When it comes to Facebook, what rewards do you get when you check it? Maybe you feel entertained by it, or perhaps it helps you feel connected with friends.

3. **Replace your habit with a different, healthier routine that maintains the same trigger and reward.** For example, let's say boredom tends to trigger your Facebook habit, and logging on helps you feel more connected to your friends. A healthier habit might be to take a quick break from work to walk outside and send a friend a personal message.

# Daily Gratitude

Use the daily gratitude worksheet to record moments for which you're thankful. Be specific, and try to notice something new and different every day, so that your mind stays alert for new reasons to be grateful.

Use the habit tracker on page 31 to mark the days when you succeed in maintaining healthy habits. Keep the list of habits reasonable and realistic, and track them for at least 30 days before moving on to new habits.

| | |
|---|---|
| **M** | *I am thankful for the 10-minute walk I was able to enjoy on my lunch break.* |
| **T** | |
| **W** | |
| **TH** | |
| **F** | |
| **S** | |
| **SU** | |
| **M** | |
| **T** | |
| **W** | |
| **TH** | |
| **F** | |
| **S** | |
| **SU** | |

# Habit Tracker

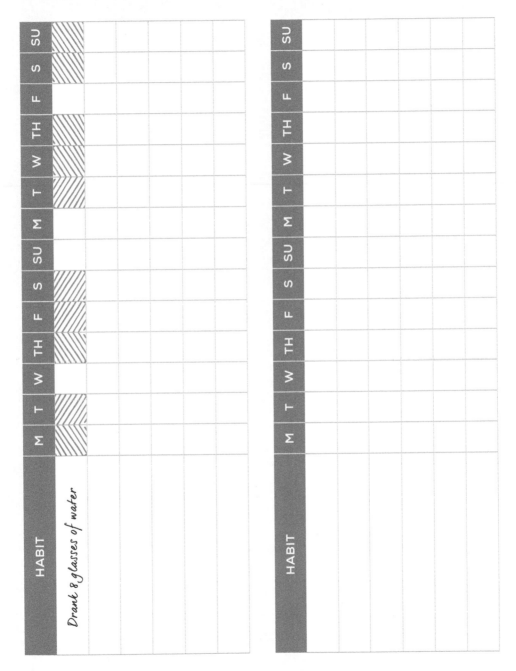

| HABIT | M | T | W | TH | F | S | SU | M | T | W | TH | F | S | SU | M | T | W | TH | F | S | SU |
|---|---|---|---|---|---|---|---|---|---|---|---|---|---|---|---|---|---|---|---|---|---|
| Drank 8 glasses of water | | | | | | | | | | | | | | | | | | | | | |
| | | | | | | | | | | | | | | | | | | | | | |
| | | | | | | | | | | | | | | | | | | | | | |
| | | | | | | | | | | | | | | | | | | | | | |
| | | | | | | | | | | | | | | | | | | | | | |

| HABIT | M | T | W | TH | F | S | SU | M | T | W | TH | F | S | SU | M | T | W | TH | F | S | SU |
|---|---|---|---|---|---|---|---|---|---|---|---|---|---|---|---|---|---|---|---|---|---|
| | | | | | | | | | | | | | | | | | | | | | |
| | | | | | | | | | | | | | | | | | | | | | |
| | | | | | | | | | | | | | | | | | | | | | |
| | | | | | | | | | | | | | | | | | | | | | |
| | | | | | | | | | | | | | | | | | | | | | |

- *Create a calm environment and a comfortable temperature.* A quiet, cool, dark environment can help you sleep better. You might consider using blackout curtains or a white noise machine to improve your sleep.

- *Sleep until the sun comes up.* Your body's internal clock will reset itself each day and help you get the best night's rest.

If you feel as if you have tried everything under the sun and nothing seems to work, then consider visiting a sleep specialist. Do whatever you need to do to manage your sleep, so you can manage your lupus.

## EXERCISE AND STRETCHING

For people with lupus, the benefits of exercising and stretching are endless. Just for starters, exercising and stretching can help reduce joint pain, improve flexibility and coordination, relieve stress, fight depression, and improve self-esteem. However, your lupus symptoms might be so uncomfortable and exhausting that it's hard to get motivated to exercise. Here are some tips to help you get started with a new exercise routine:

- *Pick the time of day that works best for you.* Although it's a good idea to get your joints moving in the morning when they are stiff, you might not be a morning person. If that's the case, exercise in the afternoon instead, or break it up into small increments throughout the day. It doesn't matter what time of day works for you, as long as you commit and do it.

- *Start out slow and know your limits.* Tailor your goals to your physical capabilities. It may be hard for you to walk right now, so consider doing water aerobics or riding a stationary bike. You might want to look into consulting an exercise therapist to help you set up a simple exercise routine and realistic goals.

- *Stretching can help you both physically and mentally.* Lupus inflammation can cause tight, stiff joints, making it difficult to get out of bed and get moving. Stretching not only helps reduce joint pain, but also improves mental health, muscle tone, and flexibility. Start with a beginner's yoga routine or 10 minutes of light stretching each morning, and build your routine from there.

- *Think of some fun activities.* Why not take up gardening, dancing, hiking, yoga, or biking? Try to approach your daily activities as a good opportunity to be active.

- *Make an effort to start weight training.* If you are taking corticosteroids to manage your lupus symptoms, keep in mind that these medications deplete the body's main bone booster, calcium. Weight training strengthens bones and can prevent fractures and osteoporosis. Start with lighter weights, such as two- to five-pound dumbbells, at least twice a week. (If you do not have weights, you can use household items such as cans of soup.)

- *Protect yourself from the sun.* It feels good to exercise out in nature, but be smart. Photosensitivity is an issue for people with lupus, and being out in the sun without proper protection or covering can lead to a flare. Invest in moisture-wicking sun-protective clothing and use a good sunscreen when exercising outside.

Before beginning any new exercise routine, discuss it with your doctor. It's important to know your limitations so you don't overdo it and cause further discomfort.

## JOY AND PLEASURE

Enjoying life when you have lupus can sometimes feel difficult, but it is definitely possible! Try to minimize some of the stress in your life to help you find happiness in the things you once enjoyed. Don't let lupus or stress diminish your joy. Let your cup run over with things that give you pleasure. Try these tips for managing stress and staying happy:

- *Savor neutral and positive experiences.* Our brains are wired to notice (and remember) negative experiences more than neutral or positive experiences—a phenomenon called negativity bias. To combat this tendency, try to note neutral or positive moments in your day and savor them for at least 6 to 12 seconds, which is the average length of time required for an experience to enter our long-term memory. Consider making a list of good things in your life you can refer to when you start to feel gloomy.

- *Seek out a support group.* A support group can give you a sense of connection, help you cope with the disease, motivate you, and provide meaningful friendship. The Resources section (page 204) lists the websites of online and local support groups throughout the country.

- *Give thanks.* No matter how you feel, start each day by writing down one or more things you are thankful for. This exercise will also help with positive thinking even in times of pain. The Daily Gratitude and Habit Trackers (pages 30 to 31) can be simple but powerful tools for cultivating gratitude.

- *Repeat a positive quotation or mantra.* This constant reminder will help you stay on top of the positive aspects of your life and approach each day as an opportunity to choose joy.

- *Explore spirituality and meditation.* Developing your spiritual side can provide a sense of hope and help you cope with illness, pain, and stress. Some studies indicate that those who describe themselves as spiritual tend to have a more positive outlook and a better quality of life. Meditation can help drown out the internal and external "noise" in our lives and let us focus on the peace and calm.

# LOVING YOUR BODY—AND YOURSELF

**Loving yourself may be the hardest part of having lupus. The visible effects of lupus can be overwhelming and can bring up feelings of anger, frustration, and shame. While it is important to acknowledge these emotions, you should not dwell on them.**

Remember that you can still be positive and productive. I can remember a few days of feeling sorry for myself, lying on the carpet of my living room and crying, "Why me?" I have done chemo three times and have gone bald three times, and my health and hair always came back. Each time it was important for me to choose to love myself, to remember who I was and what I could still accomplish. If you are suffering with hair loss, weight gain, skin rashes, and pain, it can be hard to appreciate your body and accept the things that are beyond your control. But nurturing a good relationship with who you are and loving yourself and your body will help you overcome the physical, psychological, and emotional challenges you face with lupus. There will always be challenging days when things do not go your way, but then you will have days that help you forget yesterday even happened. Instead of thinking of lupus as the end, consider it the

beginning of a new journey. Choose to love who you are, and embrace the lupus journey as an opportunity to learn and grow. If you remember one thing from this book, remember this: *Lupus does not have to define you.* You define you. You are a unique individual who just happened to get lupus. If you are struggling with depression, it is critical that you discuss this with a close friend, family member, or trained therapist, or consider calling a help line or joining a support group.

## Cultivating a Greater Love for Yourself

- **Start your day by loving yourself and choosing joy.** Remind yourself each day that you are worthy of existing and being loved. If this is hard at first, that's okay—fake it until you eventually make it.

- **Try nourishing activities that strengthen your self-compassion muscle.** Do things that help you feel relaxed and happy any time you experience suffering. Whether it's hugging a loved one for 30 seconds after a long day at work or dancing alone in your bedroom to shake the blues, learning to practice self-compassion in your daily life will build resilience for when times get tough.

- **Enjoy life-enhancing activities and exercise.** Find an exercise or physical activity that you enjoy. Exercise releases endorphins that make you feel happy.

- **Work on personal and spiritual development and live in appreciation.** Appreciate your beauty, talents, and intelligence. Find acceptance and love in your imperfections and cherish your connections to your family, friends, community, and everyone else who appreciates you for who you are.

- **Own your potential.** Spend some time considering your strengths and focusing on your positive traits. Write these down and review them regularly. Learn to love what you can still do.

- **Be patient with yourself when you are trying to change.** Life is not a race, and we all move forward at a different pace. Comparing yourself to others (or to yourself before lupus) is rarely helpful and may even damage your self-esteem.

- **Do what honors and respects you.** Avoid participating in activities that bring you down or being around people who are negative. We all have needs, and there is no shame in taking care of them.

- **Accept uncertainty and live in the moment.** Don't dwell on the past— appreciate the lessons you learned and then let it go. Life is uncertain, so try to focus on the present moment. You will be better equipped for what happens in the future if you can leave the past behind.

- **Forgive yourself.** Practice self-compassion by acknowledging that you are human and will sometimes make mistakes. Be as kind to yourself as you would be to a beloved friend in a similar situation.

- **Get support from others.** Find an online or local support group. If necessary, don't hesitate to seek professional help from a therapist or counselor.

Refer to some of my favorite resources on page 204 for more information regarding online or local support groups and education tools. Educate yourself, stay confident, and don't let lupus keep you down!

Apple Blueberry Crumble, p. 189

# 3

# Four Weeks of Smart Eating

How you eat affects how you feel more than many people understand. With these eating plans, which contain nutrients and foods beneficial for lupus, kidney conditions, heart conditions, stronger bones, and fighting inflammation, the goal isn't to overcome chronic inflammation within 28 days, but rather to help you get used to a new way of eating and living that will ultimately help you heal inflammation and even potentially send you into remission.

# Eating Mindfully

Paying attention to what you eat while you eat it may seem like a pretty basic idea on the surface, but it's surprising how few people are actually mindful as they eat. In today's fast-paced society, it's not uncommon to scarf down a meal while you're in the car, at your desk at the office, or parked in front of the television—and barely notice that you ate at all.

However, a return to mindful eating—that is, paying attention to the tastes, textures, smells, and sounds of the food as you consume it, and making the actual eating of a meal the focus of mealtime—can help you learn to experience food on a new level while noticing your body's cues for hunger, thirst, and satiation. Learning to listen to your body's signals is an important part of overall healing, not just in terms of eating but also regarding its need for rest or sleep, activity, pleasure, and the myriad other signals your body sends you daily.

Every day of your life, your body has shown up for you in numerous ways. Your legs support you as you stand. Your body digests food as you eat it and absorbs the nutrients you need. Your hands perform tasks for you. Your ears bring you the pleasure of music, and your eyes show you the beauty of scenery around you. Throughout your life, your body has been the constant and stable companion for your mind and spirit.

However, when faced with chronic illness, many tune out their body's signals because some of the feedback they receive is unpleasant.

For someone who is chronically ill, it becomes easy to ignore your body and focus mostly on mental, spiritual, and emotional stimuli instead. However, the longer you ignore your body's signals, the louder and less pleasant those signals become.

While this response is understandable, if you are unable or unwilling to listen to your body's signals, healing becomes much more difficult. Your body—even a body with chronic illness—is the expert on what it needs, so it's important to listen to it. As you begin to tune in to your body's signals again through the process of mindful eating, you'll begin to respond to what it asks for: to eat when it is hungry, to stop eating when it is full, to give it certain health-promoting foods, to rest when it is tired, to move when it craves movement, and more.

Here are some tips to help you practice mindful eating:

- Set aside a time just for eating. Turn off the television and avoid other distractions.

- Before you start to eat, notice the food. Notice its texture, colors, shapes, and aromas. Make eating a satisfying sensory experience.

- As you eat, notice how the flavors of the food change as you chew it, how it feels in your mouth, and how it feels as it travels down your throat into your stomach.

- Pay attention and listen as your body asks you to eat more, to stop eating when it's satisfied, and to drink when it is thirsty.

# The Basic Lupus Diet Meal Plan

What follows is a basic meal plan for those who have lupus without other complications like cardiovascular or kidney disease. This is a basic anti-inflammatory diet for people who can tolerate some of the big eight allergens, nightshades, and so on. (See the following sections for meal plans tailored toward those with specific complicating conditions.)

The plan that follows is a four-week plan for two people, and weekly shopping lists for the meal plan can be found in Appendix A (page 209). All the recipes provide four or more servings, so they are designed to serve two at the first meal and then be served again later in the week. If meals aren't used for leftovers, most can be stored in the freezer for use in the coming weeks and months. Storing leftovers to eat on another day saves time and energy, which is particularly welcome when you are experiencing a flare-up of your lupus.

## WEEK 1

### MONDAY

**Breakfast:** Chocolate-Banana Smoothie
**Lunch:** New England Clam Chowder
**Dinner:** Stuffed Portobello Mushrooms
**Snack Suggestions:** hardboiled eggs; Roasted Pumpkin Seeds; ½ banana

### TUESDAY

**Breakfast:** Hot Cereal with Dried Fruit
**Lunch:** Cobb Salad
**Dinner:** Easy Tuna Casserole and Almond Meal Biscuits with Honey
**Snack Suggestions:** ½ cup blueberries with ½ cup plain yogurt; Roasted Pumpkin Seeds; Ambrosia Salad

### WEDNESDAY

**Breakfast:** Easy Granola
**Lunch:** leftover New England Clam Chowder
**Dinner:** Turkey Burgers, Protein Style and tossed salad with Ginger-Garlic Vinaigrette
**Snack Suggestions:** leftover Ambrosia Salad; ½ avocado with 2 tablespoons Roasted Pumpkin Seeds; carrot sticks with Zucchini Hummus

### THURSDAY

**Breakfast:** Avocado and Berry Smoothie
**Lunch:** leftover Easy Tuna Casserole
**Dinner:** Hearty Vegetable and Lentil Soup
**Snack Suggestions:** Pumpkin Pie Smoothie; carrot and celery sticks with 2 tablespoons almond butter; ½ cup plain yogurt with dried apples

### FRIDAY

**Breakfast:** leftover Easy Granola
**Lunch:** leftover Hearty Vegetable and Lentil Soup
**Dinner:** Broccoli Beef Stir-Fry and Cauliflower Rice
**Snack Suggestions:** carrot sticks with Zucchini Hummus; ½ banana, sliced, with ½ cup plain yogurt; Almond, Flax, and Chocolate Smoothie

### SATURDAY

**Breakfast:** Blueberry Pancakes
**Lunch:** Asparagus Quiche
**Dinner:** Pork Chops and Applesauce
**Snack Suggestions:** Quick Hot Chocolate;
Sesame Kale Chips; hardboiled eggs

### SUNDAY

**Breakfast:** Swiss Chard Frittata
**Lunch:** Tuna Melt
**Dinner:** Salmon and Summer Squash
**Snack Suggestions:** Ambrosia Salad; apple
slices with 2 tablespoons almond butter;
Sesame Kale Chips

## WEEK 2

### MONDAY

**Breakfast:** Easy Granola
**Lunch:** Egg Salad
**Dinner:** White Bean Chili
**Snack Suggestions:** ½ cup plain yogurt
with ½ cup blueberries; Baked Sweet Potato
Wedges; jicama slices with salsa

### TUESDAY

**Breakfast:** Chocolate-Banana Smoothie
**Lunch:** leftover Egg Salad
**Dinner:** Chicken Noodle Soup
**Snack Suggestions:** sliced apples and almond
butter; Green Smoothie with Berries;
½ banana, sliced, with ½ cup plain yogurt

### WEDNESDAY

**Breakfast:** leftover Easy Granola
**Lunch:** leftover White Bean Chili
**Dinner:** Quick Chicken and Broccoli Stir-Fry
and Cauliflower Rice
**Snack Suggestions:** Baked Sweet Potato
Wedges; ¼ avocado with 2 tablespoons
pumpkin seeds; 1 apple

### THURSDAY

**Breakfast:** Hot Cereal with Dried Fruit
**Lunch:** leftover Chicken Noodle Soup
**Dinner:** Sirloin Steak with Chimichurri and
tossed salad with Lemon-Basil Vinaigrette
**Snack Suggestions:** 1 pear; Almond, Flax,
and Chocolate Smoothie; 1 ounce almonds

### FRIDAY

**Breakfast:** Bacon and Egg Scramble
**Lunch:** Shrimp Salad in Avocado Halves
**Dinner:** Baked White Fish with Mango Salsa
**Snack Suggestions:** Spiced Walnuts;
hardboiled egg; Citrus Berry Fizz

### SATURDAY

**Breakfast:** Anti-Inflammatory Eggs Benedict
**Lunch:** leftover Sirloin Steak with Chimichurri
**Dinner:** Meatloaf with Sweet and Sour Glaze
and Roasted Brussels Sprouts
**Snack Suggestions:** Spiced Walnuts;
½ apple with 2 tablespoons almond butter;
1 Date Bonbon

### SUNDAY

*Breakfast:* Turkey Breakfast Sausage and Sweet Potato Hash Browns
*Lunch:* Warm Spinach Salad with Shrimp
*Dinner:* Asian Salmon with Spicy Coleslaw
*Snack Suggestions:* 1 Date Bonbon; 1 pear; Avocado, Banana, and Kale Smoothie

## WEEK 3

### MONDAY

*Breakfast:* Hot Cereal with Dried Fruit
*Lunch:* leftover Asian Salmon with Spicy Coleslaw
*Dinner:* Turkey Piccata with Zucchini Noodles
*Snack Suggestions:* 1 Date Bonbon; ½ cup plain yogurt with ½ banana, sliced; Zucchini Hummus with sliced red bell peppers

### TUESDAY

*Breakfast:* Bacon and Egg Scramble
*Lunch:* Taco Soup
*Dinner:* Cod and Chickpea Packets
*Snack Suggestions:* Pumpkin Pie Smoothie; ½ apple with 2 tablespoons almond butter; 1 ounce almonds

### WEDNESDAY

*Breakfast:* Chocolate-Banana Smoothie
*Lunch:* leftover Turkey Piccata with Zucchini Noodles
*Dinner:* Bacon-Wrapped Rosemary Chicken Drumsticks with Creamy Avocado Coleslaw
*Snack Suggestions:* Zucchini Hummus with sliced red bell peppers; 1 Date Bonbon; ¼ avocado with 2 tablespoons pumpkin seeds

### THURSDAY

*Breakfast:* Easy Granola
*Lunch:* leftover Taco Soup
*Dinner:* Coconut Fish Curry and Cauliflower Rice
*Snack Suggestions:* ½ cup plain yogurt with 1 tablespoon flaxseed meal, and ½ cup blueberries; 1 Easy Almond Butter Cookie; jicama slices with salsa

### FRIDAY

*Breakfast:* Avocado and Berry Smoothie
*Lunch:* leftover Coconut Fish Curry
*Dinner:* Mustard-Rubbed Pork Tenderloin with Warm Fruit Compote and Sweet Potato Purée
*Snack Suggestions:* Avocado, Banana, and Kale Smoothie; Zucchini Hummus with sliced red bell peppers; ½ banana

### SATURDAY

*Breakfast:* Swiss Chard Frittata
*Lunch:* leftover Mustard-Rubbed Pork Tenderloin with Warm Fruit Compote and Sweet Potato Purée
*Dinner:* Easy Roasted Chicken and Balsamic-Glazed Mixed Vegetables
*Snack Suggestions:* Chocolate-Covered Frozen Banana; carrot sticks with 2 tablespoons almond butter; ½ banana, sliced, with 1 tablespoon honey and ¼ cup almond milk

**Breakfast:** Blueberry Pancakes
**Lunch:** leftover Easy Roasted Chicken and Balsamic-Glazed Mixed Vegetables
**Dinner:** Mushroom Stroganoff and Zucchini Noodles
**Snack Suggestions:** Chocolate-Covered Frozen Banana; Green Smoothie with Berries; ½ cup unsweetened applesauce

## WEEK 4

### MONDAY

**Breakfast:** Easy Granola
**Lunch:** leftover Mushroom Stroganoff and Zucchini Noodles
**Dinner:** Fish and Chips
**Snack Suggestions:** Sesame Kale Chips; ¼ avocado with 2 tablespoons pumpkin seeds; ½ cup plain yogurt with ½ banana

### TUESDAY

**Breakfast:** Bacon and Egg Scramble
**Lunch:** Butternut Squash Soup
**Dinner:** Fried Egg on a Bed of Sautéed Kale
**Snack Suggestions:** Zucchini Hummus with carrot sticks; hardboiled egg; Chia Vanilla Milk Shake; 1 ounce almonds

### WEDNESDAY

**Breakfast:** Hot Cereal with Dried Fruit
**Lunch:** leftover Fish and Chips
**Dinner:** Shrimp Scampi on Zucchini Noodles
**Snack Suggestions:** Sesame Kale Chips; hardboiled egg; ½ apple with 2 tablespoons almond butter

### THURSDAY

**Breakfast:** Avocado and Berry Smoothie
**Lunch:** leftover Butternut Squash Soup
**Dinner:** Turkey and Green Bean Packets
**Snack Suggestions:** Zucchini Hummus with carrot sticks; hardboiled egg; ½ cup plain yogurt with ½ cup blueberries

### FRIDAY

**Breakfast:** Easy Granola
**Lunch:** leftover Shrimp Scampi on Zucchini Noodles
**Dinner:** White Fish and Stone Fruit Packets
**Snack Suggestions:** Green Smoothie with Berries; jicama slices with salsa; low-sodium turkey jerky; 1 apple with 2 tablespoons almond butter

### SATURDAY

**Breakfast:** Anti-Inflammatory Eggs Benedict
**Lunch:** leftover Turkey and Green Bean Packets
**Dinner:** Mexican Black Bean Stew
**Snack Suggestions:** roasted chickpeas; Orange Creamsicle Smoothie; carrot sticks with Honey Mustard Dressing

### SUNDAY

**Breakfast:** Blueberry Pancakes
**Lunch:** leftover White Fish and Stone Fruit Packets
**Dinner:** Orange-Honey Glazed Salmon
**Snack Suggestions:** low-sodium turkey jerky; jicama slices with salsa; ½ cup plain yogurt with 1 tablespoon flaxseed meal and ½ banana, sliced

# The Flare Soother Meal Plan

Meals in the Flare Soother meal plan have lots of anti-inflammatory properties. Most are also free of ingredients that may exacerbate inflammation, like the big eight allergens and nightshades. Please follow any "Flare Soother" tips provided with the recipes, which will offer suggestions for boosting the inflammation-fighting properties of a recipe, and please follow any "Fatigue-Friendly" recipe tips, which will offer suggestions on how to prepare the meal more easily when you're feeling exhausted or suffering a lot of pain. If you are allergic to fish or shellfish, replace any seafood meal with another meal labeled "Flare Soother."

The plan that follows is a four-week plan for two people, and weekly shopping lists for the meal plan can be found in Appendix A (page 209). All the recipes provide four or more servings, so they are designed to serve two at the first meal and then be served again later in the week. If meals aren't used for leftovers, most can be stored in the freezer for use in the coming weeks and months. Storing leftovers to eat on another day saves time and energy, which is particularly welcome when you are experiencing a flare-up of your lupus.

## WEEK 1

### MONDAY

*Breakfast:* Chocolate-Banana Smoothie
*Lunch:* New England Clam Chowder
*Dinner:* Stuffed Portobello Mushrooms
*Snack Suggestions:* hardboiled eggs; Roasted Pumpkin Seeds; ½ banana

### TUESDAY

*Breakfast:* Hot Cereal with Dried Fruit
*Lunch:* Cobb Salad
*Dinner:* Easy Tuna Casserole and tossed salad with Lemon-Basil Vinaigrette
*Snack Suggestions:* ½ cup blueberries with ½ cup plain yogurt; Roasted Pumpkin Seeds; Ambrosia Salad

### WEDNESDAY

*Breakfast:* plain yogurt parfait made with raspberries, flaxseed meal, and honey
*Lunch:* leftover New England Clam Chowder
*Dinner:* Turkey Burgers, Protein Style and tossed salad with Ginger-Garlic Vinaigrette
*Snack Suggestions:* Ambrosia Salad; ½ avocado with 2 tablespoons Roasted Pumpkin Seeds; carrot sticks with Zucchini Hummus

### THURSDAY

*Breakfast:* Avocado and Berry Smoothie
*Lunch:* leftover Easy Tuna Casserole
*Dinner:* Hearty Vegetable and Lentil Soup
*Snack Suggestions:* Pumpkin Pie Smoothie; carrot and celery sticks with Zucchini Hummus; ½ cup plain yogurt with sliced apples

### FRIDAY

*Breakfast:* Pumpkin Pie Smoothie
*Lunch:* leftover Hearty Vegetable and Lentil Soup
*Dinner:* Broccoli Beef Stir-Fry and Cauliflower Rice
*Snack Suggestions:* carrot sticks with Zucchini Hummus; ½ banana, sliced, with ½ cup plain yogurt; Ginger-Lemon Tea

### SATURDAY

*Breakfast:* Blueberry Pancakes
*Lunch:* Asparagus Quiche
*Dinner:* Pork Chops and Applesauce
*Snack Suggestions:* Quick Hot Chocolate; Sesame Kale Chips; hardboiled eggs

### SUNDAY

*Breakfast:* Swiss Chard Frittata
*Lunch:* Tuna Melt
*Dinner:* Salmon and Summer Squash
*Snack Suggestions:* Ambrosia Salad; 1 apple; Sesame Kale Chips

## WEEK 2

### MONDAY

*Breakfast:* Green Smoothie with Berries
*Lunch:* salad greens with 3 ounces rotisserie chicken and 2 tablespoons Ginger-Garlic Vinaigrette
*Dinner:* White Bean Chili
*Snack Suggestions:* ½ cup plain yogurt with ½ cup blueberries; Baked Sweet Potato Wedges; 1 pear

### TUESDAY

*Breakfast:* Chocolate-Banana Smoothie
*Lunch:* leftover White Bean Chili
*Dinner:* Chicken Noodle Soup
*Snack Suggestions:* 1 apple; Green Smoothie with Berries; ½ banana, sliced, with ½ cup plain yogurt

### WEDNESDAY

*Breakfast:* Green Smoothie with Berries
*Lunch:* 2 cups Vegetable Broth with 1 cup peas
*Dinner:* Quick Chicken and Broccoli Stir-Fry and Cauliflower Rice
*Snack Suggestions:* Baked Sweet Potato Wedges; ¼ avocado with 2 tablespoons pumpkin seeds; 1 apple

### THURSDAY

*Breakfast:* Hot Cereal with Dried Fruit
*Lunch:* leftover Chicken Noodle Soup
*Dinner:* Sirloin Steak with Chimichurri and a green salad with Lemon-Basil Vinaigrette
*Snack Suggestions:* 1 pear; Orange Creamsicle Smoothie; 1 ounce pumpkin seeds

### FRIDAY

*Breakfast:* Bacon and Egg Scramble
*Lunch:* Shrimp Salad in Avocado Halves
*Dinner:* Baked White Fish with Mango Salsa
*Snack Suggestions:* 1 ounce pumpkin seeds; 1 hardboiled egg; Citrus Berry Fizz

### SATURDAY

*Breakfast:* Anti-Inflammatory Eggs Benedict
*Lunch:* leftover Sirloin Steak with Chimichurri
*Dinner:* Meatloaf with Sweet and Sour Glaze and Roasted Brussels Sprouts
*Snack Suggestions:* 1 ounce sunflower or pumpkin seeds; 1 apple; 1 Date Bonbon

## SUNDAY

*Breakfast:* Turkey Breakfast Sausage and Sweet Potato Hash Browns
*Lunch:* Sweet Potato Curry
*Dinner:* Asian Salmon with Spicy Coleslaw
*Snack Suggestions:* 1 Date Bonbon; 1 pear; Avocado, Banana, and Kale Smoothie

## WEEK 3

### MONDAY

*Breakfast:* Hot Cereal with Dried Fruit
*Lunch:* leftover Asian Salmon with Spicy Coleslaw
*Dinner:* Turkey Piccata with Zucchini Noodles
*Snack Suggestions:* 1 Date Bonbon; ½ cup plain yogurt with ½ banana, sliced; Zucchini Hummus with carrot sticks

### TUESDAY

*Breakfast:* Bacon and Egg Scramble
*Lunch:* Taco Soup
*Dinner:* Cod and Chickpea Packets
*Snack Suggestions:* Pumpkin Pie Smoothie; 1 apple; 1 ounce sunflower or pumpkin seeds

### WEDNESDAY

*Breakfast:* Chocolate-Banana Smoothie
*Lunch:* leftover Turkey Piccata with Zucchini Noodles
*Dinner:* Bacon-Wrapped Rosemary Chicken Drumsticks with Creamy Avocado Coleslaw
*Snack Suggestions:* Zucchini Hummus with carrot sticks; 1 Date Bonbon; ¼ avocado with 2 tablespoons pumpkin seeds

### THURSDAY

*Breakfast:* yogurt parfait made with ½ cup plain yogurt, 1 cup raspberries, and 2 tablespoons flaxseed meal
*Lunch:* leftover Taco Soup
*Dinner:* Coconut Fish Curry and Cauliflower Rice
*Snack Suggestions:* ½ cup plain yogurt with 1 tablespoon flaxseed meal, and ½ cup blueberries; celery sticks with Zucchini Hummus

### FRIDAY

*Breakfast:* Avocado and Berry Smoothie
*Lunch:* leftover Coconut Fish Curry and Cauliflower Rice
*Dinner:* Mustard-Rubbed Pork Tenderloin with Warm Fruit Compote and Sweet Potato Purée
*Snack Suggestions:* Avocado, Banana, and Kale Smoothie; Zucchini Hummus with carrot sticks; ½ banana

### SATURDAY

*Breakfast:* Swiss Chard Frittata
*Lunch:* leftover Mustard-Rubbed Pork Tenderloin with Warm Fruit Compote and Sweet Potato Purée
*Dinner:* Easy Roasted Chicken and Balsamic-Glazed Mixed Vegetables
*Snack Suggestions:* Chocolate-Covered Frozen Banana; carrot sticks; ½ banana, sliced, with 1 tablespoon honey and ¼ cup lite coconut milk

## SUNDAY

**Breakfast:** Blueberry Pancakes
**Lunch:** leftover Easy Roasted Chicken and Balsamic-Glazed Mixed Vegetables
**Dinner:** Mushroom Stroganoff and Zucchini Noodles
**Snack Suggestions:** Chocolate-Covered Frozen Banana; Green Smoothie with Berries; ½ cup unsweetened applesauce

## WEEK 4

### MONDAY

**Breakfast:** Chia Vanilla Milk Shake
**Lunch:** leftover Mushroom Stroganoff and Zucchini Noodles
**Dinner:** Turkey and Green Bean Packets
**Snack Suggestions:** Sesame Kale Chips; ¼ avocado with 2 tablespoons pumpkin seeds; ½ cup plain yogurt with ½ banana, sliced

### TUESDAY

**Breakfast:** Bacon and Egg Scramble
**Lunch:** Butternut Squash Soup
**Dinner:** Fried Egg on a Bed of Sautéed Kale
**Snack Suggestions:** Zucchini Hummus with carrot sticks; hardboiled egg; Chia Vanilla Milk Shake

### WEDNESDAY

**Breakfast:** Hot Cereal with Dried Fruit
**Lunch:** leftover Turkey and Green Bean Packets
**Dinner:** Shrimp Scampi on Zucchini Noodles
**Snack Suggestions:** Sesame Kale Chips; hardboiled egg; 1 apple

### THURSDAY

**Breakfast:** Avocado and Berry Smoothie
**Lunch:** leftover Butternut Squash Soup
**Dinner:** Pork Chops and Applesauce
**Snack Suggestions:** Zucchini Hummus with carrot sticks; hardboiled egg; ½ cup plain yogurt with ½ cup blueberries

### FRIDAY

**Breakfast:** Pumpkin Pie Smoothie
**Lunch:** leftover Shrimp Scampi on Zucchini Noodles
**Dinner:** White Fish and Stone Fruit Packets
**Snack Suggestions:** Green Smoothie with Berries; low-sodium turkey jerky; 1 apple

### SATURDAY

**Breakfast:** Anti-Inflammatory Eggs Benedict
**Lunch:** leftover Pork Chops and Applesauce
**Dinner:** Mexican Black Bean Stew
**Snack Suggestions:** roasted chickpeas; Orange Creamsicle Smoothie; carrot sticks

### SUNDAY

**Breakfast:** Blueberry Pancakes
**Lunch:** leftover White Fish and Stone Fruit Packets
**Dinner:** Orange-Honey Glazed Salmon
**Snack Suggestions:** low-sodium turkey jerky; ½ cup plain yogurt with 1 tablespoon flaxseed meal and ½ banana, sliced; 1 pear

# The Kidney Support Meal Plan

This plan is for people who have kidney issues associated with their lupus. These recipes minimize sodium, potassium, and fat to nurture and strengthen the kidneys. Be sure to follow any Kidney Support tips at the end of each recipe as well.

The plan that follows is a four-week plan for two people, and weekly shopping lists for the meal plan can be found in Appendix A (page 209). All the recipes provide four or more servings, so they are designed to serve two at the first meal and then be served again later in the week. If meals aren't used for leftovers, most can be stored in the freezer for use in the coming weeks and months. Storing leftovers to eat on another day saves time and energy, which is particularly welcome when you are experiencing a flare-up of your lupus.

## WEEK 1

### MONDAY

*Breakfast:* Chocolate-Banana Smoothie
*Lunch:* New England Clam Chowder
*Dinner:* Stuffed Portobello Mushrooms
*Snack Suggestions:* 1 apple; Roasted Pumpkin Seeds, ½ cup plain yogurt with ¼ cup berries

### TUESDAY

*Breakfast:* Hot Cereal with Dried Fruit
*Lunch:* salad greens with 3 ounces rotisserie chicken and 2 tablespoons Lemon-Basil Vinaigrette
*Dinner:* Easy Tuna Casserole and steamed asparagus
*Snack Suggestions:* ½ cup blueberries with ½ cup plain yogurt; Roasted Pumpkin Seeds; Ambrosia Salad

### WEDNESDAY

*Breakfast:* plain yogurt parfait made with raspberries, flaxseed meal, and honey
*Lunch:* leftover New England Clam Chowder
*Dinner:* Turkey Burgers, Protein Style and tossed salad with Ginger-Garlic Vinaigrette
*Snack Suggestions:* Ambrosia Salad; jicama sticks and salsa; carrot sticks with Zucchini Hummus

### THURSDAY

*Breakfast:* Chia Vanilla Milk Shake
*Lunch:* leftover Easy Tuna Casserole
*Dinner:* Hearty Vegetable and Lentil Soup
*Snack Suggestions:* Pumpkin Pie Smoothie; carrot and celery sticks with Zucchini Hummus; ½ cup plain yogurt with sliced apples

### FRIDAY

*Breakfast:* 2 eggs, scrambled, and Sweet Potato Hash Browns
*Lunch:* leftover Hearty Vegetable and Lentil Soup
*Dinner:* Broccoli Beef Stir-Fry and Cauliflower Rice
*Snack Suggestions:* Carrot sticks with Zucchini Hummus; ½ cup raspberries with ½ cup plain yogurt; Ginger-Lemon Tea

### SATURDAY

*Breakfast:* Bacon and Egg Scramble
*Lunch:* Asparagus Quiche
*Dinner:* Pork Chops and Applesauce
*Snack Suggestions:* Quick Hot Chocolate; Sesame Kale Chips; ½ apple with 1 tablespoon almond butter

### SUNDAY

*Breakfast:* Swiss Chard Frittata
*Lunch:* Tuna Melt
*Dinner:* Salmon and Summer Squash
*Snack Suggestions:* Ambrosia Salad; 1 apple; Sesame Kale Chips

## WEEK 2

### MONDAY

*Breakfast:* Green Smoothie with Berries
*Lunch:* salad greens with 3 ounces rotisserie chicken and 2 tablespoons Ginger-Garlic Vinaigrette
*Dinner:* Zucchini Noodles with Tri-Pepper Sauce
*Snack Suggestions:* ½ cup plain yogurt with ½ cup blueberries; Baked Sweet Potato Wedges; 1 pear

### TUESDAY

*Breakfast:* Chocolate-Banana Smoothie
*Lunch:* leftover Zucchini Noodles with Tri-Pepper Sauce
*Dinner:* Chicken Noodle Soup
*Snack Suggestions:* 1 apple; Green Smoothie with Berries; ½ cup raspberries with ½ cup plain yogurt

### WEDNESDAY

*Breakfast:* Green Smoothie with Berries
*Lunch:* Spaghetti Squash Frittata
*Dinner:* Quick Chicken and Broccoli Stir-Fry and Cauliflower Rice
*Snack Suggestions:* Baked Sweet Potato Wedges; Summer Berry Salad; 1 apple

### THURSDAY

*Breakfast:* Hot Cereal with Dried Fruit
*Lunch:* leftover Chicken Noodle Soup
*Dinner:* Sirloin Steak with Chimichurri and tossed salad with Lemon-Basil Vinaigrette
*Snack Suggestions:* Summer Berry Salad; Orange Creamsicle Smoothie; 1 ounce pumpkin seeds

### FRIDAY

*Breakfast:* Bacon and Egg Scramble
*Lunch:* Shrimp Salad in Avocado Halves
*Dinner:* Baked White Fish with Mango Salsa
*Snack Suggestions:* 1 ounce pumpkin seeds; ½ apple with 1 tablespoon almond butter; Citrus Berry Fizz

### SATURDAY

**Breakfast:** Caramelized Onion Frittata
**Lunch:** leftover Sirloin Steak with Chimichurri
**Dinner:** Meatloaf with Sweet and Sour Glaze and Honey-Glazed Carrots
**Snack Suggestions:** 1 ounce sunflower or pumpkin seeds; 1 apple; 1 Date Bonbon

### SUNDAY

**Breakfast:** Turkey Breakfast Sausage and Sweet Potato Hash Browns
**Lunch:** Creamy Avocado Coleslaw with 3 ounces rotisserie chicken
**Dinner:** Red Beans and Cauliflower Rice
**Snack Suggestions:** 1 Date Bonbon; 1 pear; Chia Vanilla Milk Shake

## WEEK 3

### MONDAY

**Breakfast:** Hot Cereal with Dried Fruit
**Lunch:** leftover Red Beans and Cauliflower Rice
**Dinner:** Turkey Piccata and Zucchini Noodles
**Snack Suggestions:** 1 Date Bonbon; ½ cup plain yogurt with 1 cup strawberries; Zucchini Hummus with carrot sticks

### TUESDAY

**Breakfast:** Bacon and Egg Scramble
**Lunch:** Taco Soup
**Dinner:** Cod and Chickpea Packets
**Snack Suggestions:** Pumpkin Pie Smoothie; 1 apple; 1 ounce sunflower or pumpkin seeds

### WEDNESDAY

**Breakfast:** Almond, Flax, and Chocolate Smoothie
**Lunch:** leftover Turkey Piccata and Zucchini Noodles
**Dinner:** Bacon-Wrapped Rosemary Chicken Drumsticks with tossed salad and 2 tablespoons Ginger-Garlic Vinaigrette
**Snack Suggestions:** Zucchini Hummus with carrot sticks; 1 Date Bonbon; 1 ounce almonds

### THURSDAY

**Breakfast:** yogurt parfait made with ½ cup plain yogurt, 1 cup raspberries, and 2 tablespoons flaxseed meal
**Lunch:** leftover Taco Soup
**Dinner:** Coconut Fish Curry and Cauliflower Rice
**Snack Suggestions:** ½ cup plain yogurt, 1 tablespoon flaxseed meal, and ½ cup blueberries; celery sticks

### FRIDAY

**Breakfast:** Avocado and Berry Smoothie
**Lunch:** leftover Coconut Fish Curry and Cauliflower Rice
**Dinner:** Mustard-Rubbed Pork Tenderloin with Warm Fruit Compote and Sweet Potato Purée
**Snack Suggestions:** Zucchini Hummus with carrot sticks; 1 ounce almonds; 1 pear

### SATURDAY

*Breakfast:* Swiss Chard Frittata
*Lunch:* leftover Mustard-Rubbed Pork Tenderloin with Warm Fruit Compote and Sweet Potato Purée
*Dinner:* Easy Roasted Chicken and Balsamic-Glazed Mixed Vegetables
*Snack Suggestions:* carrot sticks and almond butter; 1 pear; jicama sticks and salsa

### SUNDAY

*Breakfast:* 1 fried egg and Turkey Breakfast Sausage
*Lunch:* leftover Easy Roasted Chicken and Balsamic-Glazed Mixed Vegetables
*Dinner:* Mushroom Stroganoff and Zucchini Noodles
*Snack Suggestions:* Green Smoothie with Berries; ½ cup unsweetened applesauce, carrots with 1 tablespoon almond butter

## WEEK 4

### MONDAY

*Breakfast:* Chia Vanilla Milk Shake
*Lunch:* leftover Mushroom Stroganoff and Zucchini Noodles
*Dinner:* Turkey and Green Bean Packets
*Snack Suggestions:* Sesame Kale Chips; ½ cup plain yogurt with ½ banana, sliced; jicama sticks and salsa

### TUESDAY

*Breakfast:* Bacon and Egg Scramble
*Lunch:* Butternut Squash Soup
*Dinner:* Fried Egg on a Bed of Sautéed Kale
*Snack Suggestions:* Zucchini Hummus with carrot sticks; ½ cup plain yogurt with ½ cup raspberries; Chia Vanilla Milk Shake

### WEDNESDAY

*Breakfast:* Hot Cereal with Dried Fruit
*Lunch:* leftover Turkey and Green Bean Packets
*Dinner:* Shrimp Scampi on Zucchini Noodles
*Snack Suggestions:* Sesame Kale Chips; 1 apple; 1 ounce almonds

### THURSDAY

*Breakfast:* Orange Creamsicle Smoothie
*Lunch:* leftover Butternut Squash Soup
*Dinner:* Salmon and Summer Squash
*Snack Suggestions:* Zucchini Hummus with carrot sticks; ½ apple with 1 tablespoon almond butter; ½ cup plain yogurt with ½ cup blueberries

### FRIDAY

*Breakfast:* softboiled egg and ½ cup plain yogurt with ½ cup raspberries
*Lunch:* leftover Shrimp Scampi on Zucchini Noodles
*Dinner:* White Fish and Stone Fruit Packets
*Snack Suggestions:* Green Smoothie with Berries; 2 ounces pumpkin seeds; 1 apple

SATURDAY

*Breakfast:* Swiss Chard Frittata
*Lunch:* leftover Salmon and Summer Squash
*Dinner:* Mexican Black Bean Stew
*Snack Suggestions:* jicama sticks and salsa;
Orange Creamsicle Smoothie; carrot sticks

SUNDAY

*Breakfast:* Caramelized Onion Frittata
*Lunch:* leftover White Fish and Stone Fruit
Packets
*Dinner:* Orange-Honey Glazed Salmon and
Sautéed Butternut Squash
*Snack Suggestions:* ½ cup plain yogurt
with 1 tablespoon flaxseed meal and ½ cup
raspberries; 1 pear; carrot sticks and 1 table-
spoon almond butter

# Pantry Staples

Before starting the recipes in this cookbook,
it is helpful to have a number of foods ready in
your pantry and freezer. Keeping these staples
on hand makes it much easier to prepare
recipes during a busy week—or to pivot when
a recipe suggested in a meal plan doesn't suit
your individual needs.

## CANS, JARS, BAGS, AND BOXES

- Almond milk, unsweetened
- Applesauce, unsweetened
- Apples, dried
- Apricots, dried
- Artichoke hearts
- Beans, black
- Beans, kidney
- Beans, white

- Capers
- Chickpeas
- Chiles, chopped green
- Clams, chopped
- Coconut milk, lite
- Lentils
- Pickles, dill
- Tahini
- Tomatoes, chopped
- Tuna, water-packed

## FLOURS AND BAKING NEEDS

- Almond meal/almond flour
- Arrowroot powder
- Baking soda
- Chocolate, unsweetened ("baker's")
- Cocoa powder, unsweetened
- Coconut flour

## FROZEN

- Broccoli
- Butternut squash
- Carrots
- Peas
- Spinach

## NUTS AND SEEDS

- Almonds
- Almond butter
- Chia seeds
- Coconut flakes, unsweetened
- Flaxseed meal
- Pumpkin seeds
- Sesame seeds
- Walnuts

## OILS, FATS, AND ACIDS

- Lemon juice
- Lime juice
- Oil, avocado
- Oil, coconut
- Oil, extra-virgin olive
- Oil, sesame
- Vinegar, apple cider
- Vinegar, balsamic
- Vinegar, red wine
- Vinegar, rice
- Vinegar, white

## SEASONINGS

- Allspice, ground
- Basil, dried
- Chili powder
- Chipotle pepper, ground
- Cinnamon, ground
- Cloves, ground
- Coriander, ground
- Cumin, ground
- Curry powder
- Fish sauce
- Garlic powder
- Ginger, ground
- Horseradish, prepared
- Italian herbs, dried
- Marjoram, dried
- Mushrooms, dried
- Mustard, Dijon
- Nutmeg, ground
- Onion powder
- Oregano, dried
- Paprika, smoked
- Paprika, sweet
- Pepper, black, ground

- Pepper, cayenne, ground
- Peppercorns, black
- Red pepper flakes
- Rosemary, dried
- Sage, dried
- Sea salt
- Soy sauce or tamari, gluten-free, low-sodium
- Sriracha
- Tarragon, dried
- Thyme, dried
- Vanilla extract, pure

## SWEETENERS

- Honey
- Maple syrup, pure
- Stevia

# Shopping Guide

Cooking healthy, nutritious food doesn't need to be expensive. In fact, you can create most of the meals in this cookbook inexpensively. Here are some tips to help keep your costs low:

1. Use your store circular or go online to find out what's on sale. Then stock up on canned goods and frozen foods when they are on sale or whenever you find a coupon for them.

2. Use customer loyalty cards or programs that provide special savings.

3. Buy generic or store-brand items.

4. Always shop with your meal plan in mind. Create your meal plan ahead of time, and

then make a list from that of the fresh (nonpantry) items you will need. This can help you keep from being tempted by less healthy, more expensive options.

5. Don't shop when you're hungry or thirsty.

6. Buy produce in season—it's less expensive and fresher.

7. Frozen veggies are often cheaper than fresh, but compare prices to be sure.

8. Buy herbs and spices in bulk. Bulk pricing tends to be much lower than individual jars.

9. Buy meat and seafood in "family size" packages to save money, then freeze whatever you don't need right away.

10. Drink tap water instead of bottled, unless you live in an area where the water quality is poor. If you need to purchase water, you may save money by having water delivered instead of buying it by the bottle at the grocery store. If not, stock up when bottled water is on sale, or purchase a Brita filter pitcher and buy the filter cartridges in bulk.

# Essential Equipment

There are two lists of equipment in this section: equipment that you absolutely need in order to prepare the recipes in this book (most of which you probably already have), and optional equipment that can save you time and effort and make preparation and cooking more convenient.

## EQUIPMENT YOU NEED

You'll need the following when you're preparing meals at home.

### KNIVES

Good knives are absolutely essential, but they don't have to cost an arm and a leg. What's important is to keep your knives sharpened. You'll need, at the very least, a chef's knife and a paring knife, as well as a sharpening steel or a knife sharpener to keep them sharp and ready to chop, dice, and slice.

### CUTTING BOARDS

You'll need two cutting boards: one for fruits and veggies and one for meat. Plastic is great because it is inexpensive, stows away neatly, and can be sanitized in the dishwasher or in the sink with bleach.

### BASIC COOKING UTENSILS

You'll need the following utensils:
- Measuring spoons
- Measuring cups
- Vegetable peeler
- Wooden spoon
- Rubber spatula
- Offset spatula
- Whisk
- Grater (box and rasp style)
- Can opener

### POTS, PANS, AND BOWLS

You'll need the following pots, pans, and bowls:
- Rimmed baking sheet (one or two)
- Baking pans (9-by-9-inch and 9-by-13-inch)

- Roasting pan with rack
- Wire cooling rack
- Small, medium, and large saucepans
- Large stockpot
- 12-inch nonstick sauté pan or skillet
- 12-inch ovenproof sauté pan or skillet
- Small, medium, and large mixing bowls

### STORAGE ITEMS

The following items will allow you to store leftovers for later meals:
- Zip-top bags in various sizes
- Freezer containers in various sizes
- Parchment paper
- Aluminum foil
- Plastic wrap
- Labels and marking pens

### BLENDER

You'll need a countertop blender to make smoothies. It doesn't need to be expensive, although those pricey high-powered blenders often do a better job making green smoothies and crushing ice.

## EQUIPMENT THAT'S NICE TO HAVE

The following gadgets and appliances can be helpful for prepping food quickly and easily when you're experiencing a flare.

### VEGETABLE SPIRALIZER OR NOODLER

A spiralizer allows you to make "noodles" out of veggies like zucchini and sweet potato. The easiest to use is a hand-cranked model, such as the Paderno, which runs about $30. It has multiple blade sizes so you can cut different kinds of noodles, and it's easy to use.

You can also try a sharpener-style spiralizer. These are much less expensive, but are usually more difficult to use and limited in what they can do.

Finally, you can try using a julienne peeler. This requires a little bit of work on your part, but it cuts the veggies into noodle shapes just like a spiralizer does.

### FOOD PROCESSOR

Food processors run the gamut in price from about $30 to hundreds of dollars. You don't need a top-of-the-line model, as even an inexpensive food processor allows you to quickly chop veggies, make smooth sauces, and more.

### EXPRESS CHOPPER

An express chopper, like the Ninja, quickly chops veggies and saves wear and tear on your hands and arms. It costs less than $40 and is an easy way to chop lots of veggies quickly.

### CITRUS JUICER

Citrus juicers come in an array of types and price points, from about $10 to hundreds of dollars. Citrus juicers allow you to have freshly squeezed citrus juices readily available for your cooking.

### SLOW COOKER

A slow cooker is a time-saver—you can toss in raw food in the morning and come home eight hours later to a fully cooked meal. It's a great way to minimize workload for meals.

# Tips and Tricks for Success

If this is your first time trying an anti-inflammatory diet for lupus (or even if it's not), you may hit some roadblocks on the way. Try not to get discouraged, and follow these five tips to help you be successful:

1. *During flare-ups, minimize your workload.* Consider asking others for help with work like chopping, stirring, and peeling. Likewise, it may be worth your while (and the extra bit of money it may cost) to buy prechopped veggies and fruits. Fortunately, you can find many prepared veggies in salad bars, frozen food aisles, and even in the produce department at the grocery store. Use as many of these foods as possible to make your veggie prep quick and easy.

2. *Cook ahead and freeze your leftovers.* If possible, consider cooking meals when you feel well and freezing them for when you need them. You might even want to make a habit of cooking a double batch of your favorite meals and freezing half. Keeping your freezer stocked with nutritious homemade meals is a boon when you are not feeling well or when you're on the go, and it may keep you from heading out for a convenient but less-than-nutritious fast-food meal. Use single-serving freezer storage containers and label each container with the food it contains, as well as the date you put it in the freezer. Most foods can be frozen without a loss of quality for up to a year.

3. *Minimize cravings by finding ways to enjoy your favorite foods in moderation.* It may be tempting to pop a preprepared meal in the microwave or indulge in some chocolate cake. Instead, you can satisfy your craving with a healthy Almond, Flax, and Chocolate Smoothie (page 183) or Easy Chocolate Mousse (page 188). Many of the recipes in this cookbook are adaptations of favorites and can give you ideas about how to adapt other favorite foods in nutritious and anti-inflammatory ways.

4. *Add flavor to your water.* We all know drinking plain water gets boring. Here are a few ways to jazz it up:

   - Squeeze some citrus juice into a glass of seltzer.

   - Try SweetLeaf Stevia Drops in still or sparkling water. They add a little sweetness and flavor with no sugar.

   - Make Fruit-Infused Water (page 176).

   - Make a mocktail with muddled mint, a squeeze of lime, a dash stevia, and seltzer—it's a mojito without the booze or sugar.

   - Infuse hot water with herbs or ginger to make a warm herbal beverage. Steep the herbs for five minutes in boiling water. Sweeten with a little honey.

5. *Get rid of temptation.* Go through your cupboards, pantry, and refrigerator and get rid of any off-plan foods that may tempt you, then stock up on the nutritious foods recommended in the pantry shopping list on page 51.

# Part Two

# RECIPES TO SOOTHE LUPUS

The recipes in the following chapters are designed especially to fight the inflammation associated with lupus. Each recipe includes labels and tips to help you determine the right foods and ingredients for you.

**Flare Soother:** These recipes are anti-inflammatory all-stars because they are or can be made with foods and nutrients that fight inflammation, such as ginger, turmeric, berries, omega-3 fatty acids, or superfoods. They also minimize foods that contribute to inflammation during a flare, like nightshades.

**Fatigue-Friendly:** These recipes are super easy, or they can be made easier for someone experiencing a flare (or just in need of a break).

**Kidney Support:** If you have kidney damage associated with your lupus, look for these recipes, which are or can be made lower in sodium, potassium, phosphorus, fat, and protein to help support healthy kidney function.

**Cardio Care:** These recipes are helpful for people who are experiencing heart problems such as cardiovascular disease or high blood pressure. The recipes are or can be made low in fat, saturated fat, sodium, and cholesterol.

**Bone Booster:** These recipes are or can be made high in vitamin D, calcium, and/or other minerals to help support bone health and fight osteoporosis.

**Big 8 Allergen–Free:** These foods are or can be made free of the big eight allergens: wheat, eggs, fish, shellfish, soy, tree nuts, peanuts, and dairy.

**Gluten-Free:** These recipes are gluten-free for people who have celiac disease or are sensitive to gluten.

Swiss Chard Frittata, p. 70

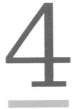

# Breakfast and Brunch

# Chocolate-Banana Smoothie

Flare Soother | Fatigue-Friendly | Kidney Support | Cardio Care | Bone Booster | Gluten-Free

A simple smoothie is a great way to make a quick, nutritious breakfast on the go with plenty of nutrients to get your day started right. One of the most appealing things about smoothies is how easy they are to customize to your own personal preferences, or to address various health conditions. You can share this smoothie with someone else or refrigerate the rest and save it for breakfast tomorrow.

**SERVES 2**
**PREP** 5 minutes
**COOK** None

2 bananas, peeled

3 tablespoons unsweetened cocoa powder

1 cup skim milk

3 tablespoons honey

½ teaspoon ground cinnamon

Pinch ground nutmeg

1 cup crushed ice

In a blender, combine all the ingredients. Blend until smooth. Pour into two tall glasses and enjoy.

Flare Soother Tip Increase the anti-inflammatory properties of this recipe by adding 2 tablespoons chia seeds or flaxseed meal, which are rich in omega-3 fatty acids. Or add ½ teaspoon ground ginger and replace 1 banana with 1 cup blueberries. Replace the skim milk, which may be inflammatory for some, with lite coconut milk.

Kidney Support Tip Replace the bananas with a lower-potassium fruit, such as 1 cup blueberries or raspberries. You can also replace the skim milk, which is relatively high in potassium, with lite coconut milk.

Big 8 Allergen Tip Replace the milk with unsweetened nut milk, such as almond milk or lite coconut milk, but remember removing the skim milk takes away the calcium boost.

PER SERVING (2 cups) Calories: 266; Carbohydrates: 64g; Protein: 7g; Cholesterol: 2mg; Total Fat: 2g; Saturated Fat: <1g; Sodium: 69mg; Potassium: 835mg; Calcium: 204mg

# Avocado and Berry Smoothie

Flare Soother | Fatigue-Friendly | Kidney Support | Cardio Care | Bone Booster | Gluten-Free

Avocados are an excellent source of vitamin E, fiber, and healthy fats. Likewise, the berries are high in antioxidants, which are excellent for fighting inflammation, and they are a flavorful source of many vitamins and minerals. This smoothie is a fantastic breakfast for when you're just not feeling great and need something you can make quickly and easily.

**SERVES 2**
**PREP** 5 minutes
**COOK** None

1 avocado, peeled and pitted

1 cup blueberries

1 cup strawberries

2 tablespoons honey

¼ teaspoon ground cloves

2 cups skim milk

1 cup crushed ice

In a blender, combine all the ingredients. Blend until smooth. Pour into two tall glasses and enjoy.

Flare Soother and Kidney Support Tip Replace the skim milk, which is relatively high in potassium and may be inflammatory for some, with lite coconut milk.

Big 8 Allergen Tip Replace the milk with unsweetened nut milk, such as almond milk or lite coconut milk, but remember removing the skim milk takes away the calcium boost.

PER SERVING (2 cups) Calories: 424; Carbohydrates: 54g; Protein: 11g; Cholesterol: 5mg; Total Fat: 20g; Saturated Fat: 4g; Sodium: 139mg; Potassium: 1,047mg; Calcium: 400mg

# Avocado, Banana, and Kale Smoothie

Flare Soother | Fatigue-Friendly | Big 8 Allergen–Free | Gluten-Free

This smoothie is loaded with delicious and nutritious anti-inflammatory ingredients that support bone strength and heart health. Avocados and bananas are both high in potassium, so if you have kidney issues it's best to avoid this recipe.

**SERVES 2**
**PREP** 5 minutes
**COOK** None

½ avocado, peeled and pitted

1 banana, peeled

2 cups stemmed kale leaves

1 cup apple juice

1 cup unsweetened nut milk such as almond milk or lite coconut milk

1 tablespoon honey

8 ice cubes

In a blender, combine all the ingredients. Blend until smooth. Serve immediately.

Cardio Care Tip  Use almond milk instead of lite coconut milk to reduce saturated fat.

Bone Booster Tip  Replace the nut milk with skim milk to boost calcium, but remember using skim milk means it is no longer allergen-free.

PER SERVING (1⅛ cups) Calories: 321; Carbohydrates: 53g; Protein: 8g; Cholesterol: 0mg; Total Fat: 10g; Saturated Fat: 2g; Sodium: 103mg; Potassium: 1,104 mg; Calcium: 300mg

# Green Smoothie with Berries

Flare Soother | Fatigue-Friendly | Kidney Support | Big 8 Allergen–Free | Gluten-Free

Spinach is a superfood that has lots of vitamins, including vitamin C and minerals. Meanwhile, berries are high in antioxidants and add sweetness to this delicious smoothie. Although it calls for raspberries, you can use any berries you choose—blackberries or blueberries are a delicious choice.

**SERVES 2**
**PREP** 5 minutes
**COOK** None

2 cups baby spinach

1 cup raspberries

1 tablespoon honey

1 cup apple juice

1 cup lite coconut milk

¼ teaspoon ground ginger

1 cup crushed ice

In a blender, combine all the ingredients. Blend until smooth. Serve immediately.

Cardio Care Tip **Use almond milk instead of lite coconut milk to reduce saturated fat.**

Bone Booster Tip **Replace the lite coconut milk with skim milk to boost calcium, but remember using skim milk means it is no longer allergen-free.**

PER SERVING (1⅛ cups) Calories: 196; Carbohydrates: 36g; Protein: 3g; Cholesterol: 0mg; Total Fat: 7g; Saturated Fat: 6g; Sodium: 60mg; Potassium: 394mg; Calcium: 72mg

# Easy Granola

Flare Soother | Fatigue-Friendly | Gluten-Free

This grain-free granola is full of nutritious omega-3 fatty acids that fight inflammation, and it has a lightly sweet flavor and lots of crunch. You can make a big batch ahead of time and keep it in an airtight container at room temperature for up to a month, which makes it the perfect breakfast for when you're having a flare-up or when you are in a hurry.

**SERVES 8**
**PREP** 10 minutes
**COOK** 25 minutes

1 cup walnuts, chopped

1 cup sliced almonds

1 cup hulled pumpkin seeds

1 cup unsweetened coconut flakes

2 tablespoons flaxseed meal

¼ cup honey

2 tablespoons coconut oil, melted

1 teaspoon pure vanilla extract

1 teaspoon ground cinnamon

¼ teaspoon ground ginger

Pinch ground nutmeg

Pinch salt

1. Preheat the oven to 300°F.

2. Line two rimmed baking sheets with parchment paper or aluminum foil.

3. In a large bowl, combine all the ingredients, mixing until well combined.

4. Spread the mixture in a single layer on each of the prepared baking sheets.

5. Bake until browned, stirring once or twice during baking, about 25 minutes. Let cool and enjoy.

Cardio Care Tip **Replace the coconut oil, which is high in saturated fat, with 2 tablespoons extra-virgin olive oil.**

PER SERVING (½ cup) Calories: 367; Carbohydrates: 18g; Protein: 11g; Cholesterol: 0mg; Total Fat: 30g; Saturated Fat: 9g; Sodium: 26mg; Potassium: 366mg; Calcium: 60mg

# Hot Cereal with Dried Fruit

Flare Soother | Fatigue-Friendly | Kidney Support | Cardio Care | Bone Booster | Gluten-Free

This is a quick and easy breakfast that doesn't involve any chopping, which makes it ideal for painful days. In fact, the only prep involved is simply measuring and stirring. This recipe is really simple to customize to your tastes and health needs because you can easily add or subtract ingredients.

**SERVES 2**
**PREP** 5 minutes
**COOK** 5 minutes

1½ cups skim milk

¼ cup coconut flour

2 tablespoons flaxseed meal

¼ cup dried apples

¼ cup dried apricots

2 tablespoons pure maple syrup

½ teaspoon ground cinnamon

1. In a small saucepan, combine all the ingredients.

2. Cook over medium heat, whisking frequently, until the mixture thickens, about 3 minutes. Serve.

Flare Soother and Big 8 Allergen Tip Replace the skim milk, which may be inflammatory for some and is an allergen, with lite coconut milk, but remember removing the skim milk takes away the calcium boost.

Kidney Support Tip Replace the dried apricots, which are high in potassium, with an equal amount of dried apples. Alternatively, stir in ½ cup fresh blueberries after the cereal is cooked. You can also replace the skim milk, which is relatively high in potassium, with lite coconut milk.

PER SERVING (½ cup) Calories: 253; Carbohydrates: 34g; Protein: 8g; Cholesterol: 4mg; Total Fat: 9g; Saturated Fat: 6g; Sodium: 106mg; Potassium: 536mg; Calcium: 400mg

# Blueberry Pancakes

Flare Soother | Fatigue-Friendly | Gluten-Free

These pancakes are the height of simplicity, containing just four ingredients and coming together in a matter of minutes. They are so tasty, easy to make, and something the entire family can enjoy together, they may just become your go-to breakfast for weekend mornings. This is also a great way to use up very ripe bananas.

**SERVES 4**
**PREP** 5 minutes
**COOK** 10 minutes

4 large eggs

2 very ripe bananas, peeled

2 tablespoons coconut flour

1 tablespoon coconut oil

1 cup frozen blueberries

½ cup pure maple syrup

1. In a blender, combine the eggs, bananas, and coconut flour to make the batter. Blend until smooth.

2. In a large, nonstick sauté pan or skillet over medium heat, heat the coconut oil until it shimmers.

3. Pour the pancake batter into the skillet in ¼-cup amounts. Sprinkle with the blueberries. Cook until bubbles form on the top, about 3 minutes. Flip the pancakes and cook until the other side is browned, a minute or two more.

4. Serve topped with the maple syrup.

**Flare Soother and Cardio Care Tip** Add 1 teaspoon ground ginger to the batter, and add 1 tablespoon chopped walnuts to each pancake when you add the blueberries. This is a great source of omega-3 fatty acids, which are good for your heart and fighting inflammation.

PER SERVING (2 pancakes, 2 tablespoons syrup) Calories: 277; Carbohydrates: 46g; Protein: 7g; Cholesterol: 164mg; Total Fat: 9g; Saturated Fat: 5g; Sodium: 66mg; Potassium: 387mg; Calcium: 60mg

# Turkey Breakfast Sausage

Flare Soother | Fatigue-Friendly | Kidney Support | Big 8 Allergen–Free | Gluten-Free

Many breakfast sausages have fillers, preservatives, and lots of sodium and saturated fat, which can cause inflammation and other issues. Try this simple, homemade turkey sausage as a side with eggs, or browned and tossed in an omelet. It's really easy to make, which is helpful when you're in a hurry or experiencing pain.

**SERVES 8**
**PREP** 10 minutes
**COOK** 10 minutes

1 pound ground
turkey breast

2 teaspoons dried sage

½ teaspoon sea salt

½ teaspoon black pepper

½ teaspoon dried thyme

⅛ teaspoon cayenne pepper

Pinch ground nutmeg

Red pepper flakes

2 tablespoons extra-virgin
olive oil

1. In a bowl, mix the ground turkey, sage, salt, pepper, thyme, cayenne, nutmeg, and red pepper flakes.

2. Form the mixture into 8 patties.

3. In a large, nonstick sauté pan or skillet over medium-high heat, heat the olive oil until it shimmers.

4. Cook the sausage patties until browned on both sides, about 3 minutes per side. Serve.

Flare Soother Tip  Red pepper flakes and cayenne are night-shades, which may contribute to inflammation in some. If you're experiencing a flare, replace these two ingredients with 1 teaspoon dried rosemary.

Kidney Support and Cardio Care Tip  Reduce the salt to ¼ teaspoon to minimize sodium intake.

PER SERVING (2-ounce patty) Calories: 139; Carbohydrates: <1g; Protein: 16g; Cholesterol: 42mg; Total Fat: 8g; Saturated Fat: 2g; Sodium: 153mg; Potassium: 169mg; Calcium: 24mg

# Anti-Inflammatory Eggs Benedict

Flare Soother | Fatigue-Friendly | Gluten-Free

Eggs benedict is a delicious and luxurious breakfast. However, the traditional recipe has ingredients that aren't heart healthy and can increase inflammation in the body. This lightened-up version eliminates many of the inflammatory ingredients while still retaining the luxurious taste and texture of the original.

**SERVES 4**
**PREP** 15 minutes
**COOK** 15 minutes

8 Canadian bacon slices

2 tablespoons white vinegar

4 large eggs

1 avocado, peeled and pitted

Grated zest and juice
of 1 lemon

1 garlic clove, minced

¼ cup water

1 tablespoon extra-virgin
olive oil

1 tablespoon walnut oil

¼ teaspoon sea salt

¼ teaspoon paprika

1. Preheat the oven to 400°F.

2. Arrange the bacon slices on a baking sheet and warm in the oven for about 10 minutes.

3. Fill a large pot with about 2 inches of water. Add the vinegar. Bring the water to a boil over medium-low heat.

4. Gently crack each of the eggs into the simmering water (see Ingredient Tip) and poach just until the whites are set, about 3 minutes.

5. Meanwhile, in a blender or food processor, combine the avocado, lemon zest and juice, garlic, water, olive oil, walnut oil, salt, and paprika. Blend until smooth.

6. To assemble, place 2 pieces of bacon on each plate. Top each with a poached egg, and spoon the sauce over the top. Serve.

Flare Soother Tip Paprika is a nightshade, which may exacerbate inflammation in some people. Eliminate it if you are sensitive to nightshades.

Fatigue-Friendly Tip Use ½ teaspoon minced garlic from a jar.

Kidney Support and Cardio Care Tip Replace the Canadian bacon with thinly sliced low-sodium cooked turkey breast to reduce sodium and saturated fat.

Ingredient Tip The best way to get the eggs into the water for poaching is to crack each egg into a custard cup. Begin swirling the water and then gently slide the egg into the water (holding the cup just above the water). Remove the cooked eggs with a slotted spoon.

PER SERVING (1 egg, 1 Canadian bacon slice, 3 tablespoons sauce) Calories: 321; Carbohydrates: 7g; Protein: 19g; Cholesterol: 192mg; Total Fat: 25g; Saturated Fat: 6g; Sodium: 985mg; Potassium: 525mg; Calcium: 48mg

# Swiss Chard Frittata

Flare Soother | Kidney Support | Bone Booster | Gluten-Free

Dark, leafy greens like Swiss chard are an excellent source of inflammation-fighting antioxidants, and they are packed with nutrition to support your overall health. Because there's minimal chopping and mixing, this is also a relatively simple meal to make when you're experiencing a flare-up of pain.

**SERVES 4**
**PREP** 5 minutes
**COOK** 15 minutes

2 tablespoons extra-virgin olive oil

2 cups Swiss chard, roughly chopped

½ red bell pepper, sliced

1 teaspoon garlic powder

½ teaspoon sea salt

⅛ teaspoon black pepper

6 eggs

2 tablespoons water

1. Heat the broiler to high heat.

2. In a large, ovenproof sauté pan or skillet over medium-high heat, heat the olive oil until it shimmers.

3. Add the Swiss chard, bell pepper, garlic powder, salt, and pepper and cook, stirring occasionally, for 5 minutes. Reduce the heat to medium.

4. In a small bowl, whisk together the eggs and the water.

5. Carefully pour the eggs over the cooked chard. Cook without stirring until the eggs begin to set around the edges, about 3 minutes.

6. Using a rubber spatula, carefully pull the solid eggs away from the edges of the pan. Tilt the pan to allow uncooked eggs to flow into the spaces you just created. Cook until eggs set again, another 1 or 2 minutes.

7. Transfer the pan to the preheated broiler. Broil until puffy and browned on top, 2 to 3 minutes. Cut into wedges to serve.

Kidney Support Tip  Moderation in the protein is key here. Reduce the serving size to ⅛ of the frittata and have a side of fresh fruit or Sweet Potato Hash Browns (page 73). Reduce salt by half to ¼ teaspoon to minimize sodium intake.

Cardio Care Tip  Use 2 whole eggs and 6 egg whites instead of 6 whole eggs to reduce fat and cholesterol. Reduce salt to ¼ teaspoon to minimize sodium.

Flare Soother Tip  Omit the red bell pepper if you are sensitive to nightshades.

Bone Booster Tip  Replace the water with ¼ cup skim milk. Add 3 tablespoons grated Parmesan cheese to the top of the frittata just before transferring it to the broiler.

PER SERVING  Calories: 165; Carbohydrates: 3g; Protein: 9g; Cholesterol: 246mg; Total Fat: 14g; Saturated Fat: 3g; Sodium: 365mg; Potassium: 165mg; Calcium: 60mg

# Bacon and Egg Scramble

Flare Soother | Fatigue-Friendly | Kidney Support | Gluten-Free

This is a great option for days when you're feeling well and want a heartier breakfast. The scramble comes together quickly and requires minimal chopping, and it offers an excellent source of protein to keep you satiated as you begin your day. It's also easy to add ingredients based on your personal preferences.

**SERVES 4**
**PREP** 10 minutes
**COOK** 10 minutes

2 tablespoons extra-virgin olive oil

4 turkey bacon slices, chopped

8 large eggs, beaten

¼ teaspoon sea salt

⅛ teaspoon black pepper

1. In a large, nonstick sauté pan or skillet over medium-high heat, heat the olive oil until it shimmers.

2. Add the bacon and cook, stirring occasionally, until browned, about 5 minutes. Reduce the heat to medium.

3. Add the eggs, salt, and pepper. Cook, stirring occasionally, until the eggs are cooked, about 4 minutes more. Serve.

Flare Soother Tip **After the bacon is cooked, add 2 cups baby spinach. Cook, stirring occasionally, until the spinach is wilted, about 3 minutes. Then proceed with the recipe as written.**

Kidney Support Tip **Halve the serving size to keep protein in check. Serve with a fruit smoothie, some fresh fruit, or Sweet Potato Hash Browns (page 73). Omit the salt and choose low-sodium bacon.**

Cardio Care Tip **Use low-sodium turkey bacon and eliminate the salt. Replace the 8 eggs with 3 whole eggs and 8 egg whites to reduce fat and cholesterol.**

PER SERVING Calories: 206; Carbohydrates: <1g; Protein: 14g; Cholesterol: 337mg; Total Fat: 16g; Saturated Fat: 4g; Sodium: 360mg; Potassium: 119mg; Calcium: 400mg

# Sweet Potato Hash Browns

Flare Soother | Fatigue-Friendly | Kidney Support | Big 8 Allergen–Free | Gluten-Free

Hash browns are a breakfast favorite for many, but potatoes are nightshades that can exacerbate inflammation in some people with autoimmune disease. Sweet potatoes are not nightshades, and they are a rich source of vitamin A, which is an anti-inflammatory nutrient.

**SERVES 2**
**PREP** 10 minutes
**COOK** 15 minutes

2 tablespoons extra-virgin olive oil

1 sweet potato, peeled and grated

½ teaspoon sea salt

¼ teaspoon black pepper

1. In a large, nonstick sauté pan or skillet over medium-high heat, heat the olive oil until it shimmers. Add the potato and sprinkle with the salt and pepper.

2. Cook without stirring until the potato browns on one side, about 7 minutes. Flip and continue cooking on the other side until browned, about 7 minutes more. Serve.

Fatigue-Friendly Tip Grating potatoes might feel like a real chore if you're experiencing a lot of pain. However, if you have a food processor, insert the shredding blade and those potatoes will be ready in seconds.

Kidney Support and Cardio Care Tip Reduce the salt to ¼ teaspoon to minimize sodium intake.

PER SERVING Calories: 172; Carbohydrates: 12g; Protein: 1g; Cholesterol: 0mg; Total Fat: 14g; Saturated Fat: 2g; Sodium: 489mg; Potassium: 274mg; Calcium: 0mg

Summer Berry Salad, p. 93

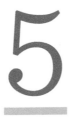

# Soups and Salads

# Avgolemono Soup with Turkey Meatballs

Fatigue-Friendly | Gluten-Free

Avgolemono is a lemon and egg soup popular in Mediterranean cuisine. This version has a bright flavor and is hearty enough to serve as your main meal. It also freezes well, so it's fantastic to make in big batches for use for when you're not feeling well or when you're simply too busy to cook.

**SERVES 4**
**PREP** 15 minutes
**COOK** 20 minutes

### FOR THE MEATBALLS

10 ounces ground
turkey breast

2 teaspoons dried rosemary

1 teaspoon dried thyme

1 teaspoon dried oregano

1 teaspoon dried marjoram

1 teaspoon garlic powder

1 teaspoon onion powder

½ teaspoon sea salt

### FOR THE SOUP

2 tablespoons extra-virgin
olive oil

1 yellow onion, chopped

2 carrots, peeled
and chopped

8 cups Chicken Broth
(page 192)

1 teaspoon garlic powder

½ teaspoon sea salt

¼ teaspoon black pepper

2 large eggs, beaten

Juice of 2 lemons

**TO MAKE THE MEATBALLS**

In a bowl, combine all the ingredients, mixing well. Form into 1-inch meatballs and set aside.

**TO MAKE THE SOUP**

1.  In a large pot over medium-high heat, heat the olive oil until it shimmers.

2.  Add the onion and cook, stirring occasionally, until soft, about 4 minutes.

3.  Add the carrots, broth, garlic powder, salt, pepper, and meatballs. Bring to a boil and then reduce the heat to medium. Cook, stirring occasionally, until the meatballs are cooked through, about 10 minutes. Remove the pot from the heat.

4.  In a small bowl, whisk together the eggs and lemon juice. In a thin stream, pour the mixture into the hot soup, stirring constantly. Serve.

Fatigue-Friendly Tip Use 1 cup each prechopped onions and carrots (fresh or frozen) from the grocery store. Mix the meatballs in a food processor until just blended, and use a small ice cream scoop or melon baller to form quick, easy meatballs.

Kidney Support and Cardio Care Tip Reduce the salt in both the meatballs and the soup to ¼ teaspoon each.

PER SERVING (3 cups) Calories: 294; Carbohydrates: 11g; Protein: 28g; Cholesterol: 134mg; Total Fat: 15g; Saturated Fat: 3g; Sodium: 710mg; Potassium: 429mg; Calcium: 204mg

# Chilled Avocado Soup

Flare Soother | Fatigue-Friendly | Big 8 Allergen–Free | Gluten-Free

This simple, tasty soup is packed with healthy fats, potassium, fiber, and vitamin E. It's also really easy to make—you can throw it together with minimal cutting and chopping and just a little blending. It's not a good make-ahead option, however, due to how quickly avocados oxidize, so plan to enjoy it right away.

**SERVES 4**
**PREP** 10 minutes
**COOK** None

2 avocados, peeled and pitted

1 garlic clove, lightly smashed

¼ cup fresh cilantro leaves

2 cups chilled lite coconut milk

Juice of 2 limes

Grated zest of 1 lime

½ teaspoon sea salt

¼ teaspoon black pepper

¼ teaspoon ground chipotle pepper

In a blender, combine all the ingredients. Blend until smooth. Serve immediately.

Flare Soother Tip **Increase the anti-inflammatory properties of this recipe by adding 1 tablespoon walnut oil, which contains omega-3 fatty acids.**

Fatigue-Friendly Tip **Instead of smashing garlic by hand, use ½ teaspoon minced garlic from a jar.**

Kidney Support and Cardio Care Tip **Moderation is key here. Reduce the serving size by half and have a salad or a serving of low-potassium fruit alongside the soup. Reduce the salt to ¼ teaspoon to minimize sodium intake.**

PER SERVING (1½ cups) Calories: 275; Carbohydrates: 14g; Protein: 4g; Cholesterol: 0mg; Total Fat: 26g; Saturated Fat: 10g; Sodium: 272mg; Potassium: 500mg; Calcium: 24mg

# Chicken Noodle Soup

Flare Soother | Fatigue-Friendly | Kidney Support | Big 8 Allergen–Free | Gluten-Free

Using grocery store rotisserie chicken meat makes this meal a snap. To make the zucchini ribbons, use a vegetable peeler to cut the zucchini into wide strips. This dish freezes well, so save individual servings in your freezer for meals on the go.

**SERVES 4**
**PREP** 15 minutes
**COOK** 15 minutes

2 tablespoons extra-virgin olive oil

1 yellow onion, chopped

2 carrots, peeled and sliced, or 1 cup frozen chopped carrots

10 cups Chicken Broth (page 192)

1 teaspoon garlic powder

1 teaspoon dried thyme

½ teaspoon sea salt

¼ teaspoon pepper

3 cups chopped rotisserie chicken

2 zucchini, cut into ribbons (see headnote)

1. In a large pot over medium-high heat, heat the olive oil until it shimmers.

2. Add the onion and fresh carrots (if using) and cook, stirring occasionally, until the vegetables start to soften, about 3 minutes.

3. Add the broth, frozen carrots (if using), garlic powder, thyme, salt, and pepper. Simmer for 5 minutes.

4. Add the chicken and zucchini ribbons. Cook for 2 minutes more to heat through. Serve.

Fatigue-Friendly Tip Some grocery stores have vegetable noodles in the produce section, such as butternut squash, zucchini, or sweet potato noodles. All of these will work well if you don't want to make your own noodles. Use 1 cup prechopped onion from the grocery store.

Kidney Support and Cardio Care Tip Reduce the salt to ¼ teaspoon to minimize sodium, and use only chicken breast meat.

PER SERVING (3 cups) Calories: 213; Carbohydrates: 12g; Protein: 20g; Cholesterol: 44mg; Total Fat: 10g; Saturated Fat: 2g; Sodium: 477mg; Potassium: 514mg; Calcium: 24mg

# Butternut Squash Soup

Flare Soother | Fatigue-Friendly | Kidney Support | Big 8 Allergen–Free | Gluten-Free

Butternut squash has a delicate, earthy flavor that's downright delicious in this silky soup. It's also full of healthy antioxidants like vitamins A and C, which can help soothe inflammation as it occurs. Make and freeze this soup for a quick meal on a busy day.

**SERVES 4**
**PREP** 15 minutes
**COOK** 10 minutes

5 cups Chicken Broth (page 192) or Vegetable Broth (page 193)

1 cup lite coconut milk

1 butternut squash, peeled and cubed

1 teaspoon onion powder

1 teaspoon garlic powder

½ teaspoon dried sage

Pinch ground nutmeg

½ teaspoon sea salt

¼ teaspoon pepper

1. In a large pot, combine all the ingredients.

2. Bring to a simmer over medium-high heat and cook, stirring occasionally, until the squash is soft, about 10 minutes.

3. Carefully transfer the soup to a countertop blender (or use an immersion blender) and purée until smooth. Serve.

Fatigue-Friendly Tip Many grocery stores offer fresh and frozen prechopped butternut squash, which you can use to replace the whole butternut squash. A 2-pound squash will yield about 3 cups of cubed squash, which is similar to the yield of a 12-ounce package of cubed squash.

Kidney Support and Cardio Care Tip Reduce the salt to ¼ teaspoon to minimize sodium content while maintaining flavor. If potassium is an issue for you, then reduce the serving size to 1 cup.

PER SERVING (2 cups) Calories: 89; Carbohydrates: 13g; Protein: 4g; Cholesterol: 0mg; Total Fat: 3g; Saturated Fat: 3g; Sodium: 340mg; Potassium: 263mg; Calcium: 24mg

# Hearty Vegetable and Lentil Soup

Flare Soother | Fatigue-Friendly | Kidney Support | Bone Booster
Big 8 Allergen–Free | Gluten-Free

Lentils serve as a nice source of protein and calcium in this soup, making it a great bone booster and an excellent vegetarian option for a hearty weeknight meal. If you use pre-chopped onions and carrots, this soup comes together in no time. Make it ahead and refrigerate for up to five days—or store in the freezer for up to a year.

**SERVES 4**
**PREP** 15 minutes
**COOK** 15 minutes

2 tablespoons extra-virgin olive oil

1 yellow onion, chopped

5 cups Vegetable Broth (page 193)

2 carrots, peeled and chopped

1 (14-ounce) can lentils, drained

1 (14-ounce) can diced tomatoes

1 teaspoon garlic powder

1 teaspoon ground turmeric

1 teaspoon dried thyme

½ teaspoon dried rosemary

½ teaspoon sea salt

¼ teaspoon black pepper

2 cups baby spinach

1. In a large pot over medium-high heat, heat the olive oil until it shimmers. Add the onion and cook, stirring occasionally, until soft, about 4 minutes.

2. Add the broth, carrots, lentils, tomatoes with their juice, garlic powder, turmeric, thyme, rosemary, salt, and pepper. Bring to a simmer. Reduce the heat to medium and simmer until the vegetables are soft, about 5 minutes.

3. Stir in the spinach. Cook until the spinach wilts, about 2 minutes more. Serve.

Flare Soother Tip Eliminate the canned tomatoes and increase the vegetable broth by 1 cup.

Fatigue-Friendly Tip Use 1 cup prechopped onion and 2 cups prechopped carrots (fresh or frozen) from the grocery store.

Kidney Support and Cardio Care Tip Replace the lentils with 1 cup frozen green peas. Reduce the salt to ¼ teaspoon to minimize sodium intake.

PER SERVING (3 cups) Calories: 488; Carbohydrates: 78g; Protein: 28g; Cholesterol: 0mg; Total Fat: 8g; Saturated Fat: 1g; Sodium: 784mg; Potassium: 1,495mg; Calcium: 84mg

# New England Clam Chowder

Flare Soother | Fatigue-Friendly | Kidney Support | Bone Booster | Gluten-Free

This creamy, fragrant clam chowder is sure to warm up any evening meal with tender veggies, aromatic herbs, and a rich and satisfying broth. Using prechopped or frozen veggies will save you time and makes for an easily prepared meal when you're dealing with a flare-up.

**SERVES 4**
**PREP** 10 minutes
**COOK** 20 minutes

2 tablespoons extra-virgin olive oil

4 turkey bacon slices, chopped

1 yellow onion, chopped

1 celery stalk, chopped

2 carrots, peeled and chopped

6 cups Chicken Broth (page 192)

2 (4-ounce) cans chopped clams

2 red potatoes, cubed

1 teaspoon dried thyme

½ teaspoon garlic powder

½ teaspoon sea salt

¼ teaspoon black pepper

2 cups skim milk

¼ cup arrowroot powder

1. In a large pot over medium-high heat, heat the olive oil until it shimmers. Add the bacon and cook, stirring occasionally, until browned, about 4 minutes. Remove the bacon with a slotted spoon and set aside on a paper towel–lined plate.

2. Add the onion, celery, and carrots to the oil remaining in the pot. Cook, stirring occasionally, until the vegetables soften, about 4 minutes.

3. Add the broth, clams with their juice, potatoes, thyme, garlic powder, salt, and pepper. Bring to a simmer and cook, stirring occasionally, until the potatoes are tender, about 10 minutes.

4. Return the bacon to the pot. In a small bowl, whisk together the milk and arrowroot powder until smooth. Add to the pot in a thin stream, stirring constantly. Cook, stirring constantly, until the soup thickens, 1 to 2 minutes more. Serve.

Flare Soother Tip Replace the potatoes, which are night-shade veggies and may exacerbate inflammation, with chopped zucchini. Replace the skim milk with an equal amount of unsweetened nut milk, but remember removing the skim milk takes away the calcium boost.

Fatigue-Friendly Tip Use 1 cup prechopped onion, 1 cup prechopped celery, and 2 cups prechopped carrots (fresh or frozen) from the grocery store. If using frozen carrots, add them in step 3 with the potatoes.

Kidney Support and Cardio Care Tip Reduce the clams to 1 can and replace the potatoes with chopped zucchini. Reduce the salt to ¼ teaspoon or eliminate it altogether, and use low-sodium bacon to minimize sodium intake.

PER SERVING (3 cups) Calories: 281; Carbohydrates: 38g; Protein: 13g; Cholesterol: 12mg; Total Fat: 8g; Saturated Fat: 1g; Sodium: 763mg; Potassium: 915mg; Calcium: 228mg

# Taco Soup

Flare Soother | Fatigue-Friendly | Kidney Support | Big 8 Allergen–Free | Gluten-Free

Instead of a traditional taco night, why not try this tasty taco soup? It's got all the Tex-Mex flavors you love, but it's super easy to prepare. It's a great meal to make ahead and freeze—if you use prechopped onions, all you have to do is open a few cans and stir.

**SERVES 4**
**PREP** 10 minutes
**COOK** 10 minutes

2 tablespoons extra-virgin olive oil

10 ounces extra-lean ground beef

1 yellow onion, chopped

1 tablespoon chili powder

1 teaspoon onion powder

1 teaspoon garlic powder

1 teaspoon dried oregano

1 teaspoon ground cumin

½ teaspoon ground coriander

½ teaspoon sea salt

⅛ teaspoon cayenne pepper

9 cups Chicken Broth (page 192)

1 (14-ounce) can diced tomatoes and green chiles (such as Ro-Tel) or 1 (14-ounce) can diced tomatoes plus 1 (2-ounce) can diced green chiles

1 (14-ounce) can black beans, rinsed and drained

1. In a large pot over medium-high heat, heat the olive oil until it shimmers. Add the ground beef and onion and cook, stirring occasionally to break up the beef, until the meat has browned, about 5 minutes.

2. Add the chili powder, onion powder, garlic powder, oregano, cumin, coriander, salt, and cayenne. Cook, stirring constantly, for 1 minute.

3. Add the broth, tomatoes and chiles with their juice, and black beans. Cook, stirring occasionally, for 3 minutes more. Serve.

Flare Soother Tip Tomatoes and chiles are nightshades and may exacerbate inflammation, so replace them with an additional cup of chicken broth. Replace the chili powder with an extra ½ teaspoon cumin, and eliminate the cayenne entirely.

Fatigue-Friendly Tip Use 1 cup prechopped onion from the grocery store.

Kidney Support Tip Reduce the ground beef to 6 ounces and reduce the black beans to half a can. Add 1 cup frozen chopped carrots when you add the chicken broth. Reduce the salt to ¼ teaspoon to minimize sodium intake.

Cardio Care Tip Replace the ground beef with ground turkey breast. Reduce the salt to ¼ teaspoon.

Bone Booster Tip Top with ¼ cup grated Monterey Jack cheese for added calcium, but remember using dairy means it is no longer allergen-free.

PER SERVING (3 cups) Calories: 587; Carbohydrates: 74g; Protein: 43g; Cholesterol: 54mg; Total Fat: 15g; Saturated Fat: 4g; Sodium: 675mg; Potassium: 1,825mg; Calcium: 228mg

# Warm Spinach Salad with Shrimp

Flare Soother | Fatigue-Friendly | Bone Booster | Gluten-Free

This delicious salad makes a tasty main course, or it's excellent as a starter course or side dish. It has a sweet-smoky dressing that perfectly complements the spinach. Spinach is high in calcium, iron, and antioxidants, so it's a powerful bone booster and flare soother.

**SERVES 4**
**PREP** 10 minutes
**COOK** 10 minutes

2 tablespoons extra-virgin olive oil

4 turkey bacon slices, chopped

2 garlic cloves, minced

¼ cup red wine vinegar

¼ cup orange juice

1 teaspoon Dijon mustard

1 teaspoon honey

½ teaspoon onion powder

½ teaspoon sea salt

⅛ teaspoon black pepper

2 (10-ounce) packages baby spinach

8 ounces cooked baby shrimp

1. In a large sauté pan or skillet over medium-high heat, heat the olive oil until it shimmers. Add the bacon and cook, stirring occasionally, until browned, about 5 minutes. Remove the bacon with a slotted spoon and set aside on a paper towel–lined plate.

2. Add the garlic, vinegar, orange juice, mustard, honey, onion powder, salt, and pepper to the pan. Bring the mixture to a simmer and cook, stirring occasionally, until the liquid reduces by half, about 4 minutes.

3. In a large bowl, combine the spinach and bacon. Pour the vinegar mixture over the top and toss. Top with the shrimp and serve.

Fatigue-Friendly Tip  Use 1 teaspoon minced garlic from a jar.

Kidney Support and Cardio Care Tip  Reduce the salt to just a pinch to minimize sodium content. Choose low-sodium bacon.

PER SERVING (about 3 cups) Calories: 177; Carbohydrates: 10g; Protein: 17g; Cholesterol: 10mg; Total Fat: 9g; Saturated Fat: 1g; Sodium: 879mg; Potassium: 845mg; Calcium: 228mg

# Chicken Caesar Salad

Flare Soother | Fatigue-Friendly | Bone Booster | Gluten-Free

Store-bought rotisserie chicken is a real time-saver when making this salad and other recipes in this book. On a day when you have a little extra time and energy, buy a whole rotisserie chicken. Remove the skin and bones and portion the meat into 4-ounce portions. Store these portions in zip-top bags in the freezer and just thaw them in the refrigerator or microwave when you're ready to use them. Reserve the bones to make Chicken Broth (page 192).

**SERVES 4**
**PREP** 10 minutes
**COOK** None

3 garlic cloves,
lightly smashed

¼ cup Easy Mayonnaise
(page 195)

1 tablespoon Dijon mustard

Grated zest and juice
of 1 lemon

½ teaspoon sea salt

¼ teaspoon black pepper

12 cups torn romaine lettuce

2 cups chopped
rotisserie chicken

1. In a blender, combine the garlic, mayonnaise, mustard, lemon zest and juice, salt, and pepper. Blend until smooth.

2. In a large bowl, combine the lettuce and chicken. Add the dressing and toss to coat. Serve.

Fatigue-Friendly Tip Use 1½ teaspoons minced garlic from a jar, and purchase pretorn, bagged lettuce for the salad.

Kidney Support and Cardio Care Tip Reduce the salt to ¼ teaspoon to minimize sodium intake. Use only chicken breast meat.

Bone Booster Tip Add ¼ cup grated Parmesan cheese to the blender to boost calcium.

PER SERVING (about 3 cups) Calories: 175; Carbohydrates: 10g; Protein: 18g; Cholesterol: 47mg; Total Fat: 7g; Saturated Fat: 1g; Sodium: 431mg; Potassium: 375mg; Calcium: 24mg

# Cobb Salad

Flare Soother | Fatigue-Friendly | Gluten-Free

You can save yourself lots of time and effort preparing this salad if you buy a rotisserie chicken, prechopped tomatoes, and bacon bits from your grocery store's salad bar. You may even be able to find packaged eggs that have already been hardboiled and peeled for you—check the refrigerated aisle (near the fresh eggs) or the deli section. While it's a little more expensive to shop this way, the convenience and ease makes it worthwhile when you're not feeling well.

**SERVES 4**
**PREP** 10 minutes
**COOK** None

10 cups torn romaine lettuce

4 large hardboiled eggs, chopped

2 cups chopped rotisserie chicken

1 cup chopped tomatoes

4 bacon slices, cooked and chopped

¼ cup Honey Mustard Dressing (page 198)

1. In a large bowl, toss together the lettuce, eggs, chicken, tomatoes, and bacon.

2. Add the dressing and toss to coat. Serve.

Flare Soother Tip **Replace the tomatoes with 1 cup diced pickled beets.**

Fatigue-Friendly Tip **Use prebagged salad mix and replace the chopped tomatoes with cherry tomatoes.**

Kidney Support Tip **Choose low-sodium bacon.**

Cardio Care Tip **Replace the bacon with turkey bacon and use only the egg whites, not the yolks.**

Bone Booster Tip **Add ¼ cup grated blue cheese for extra calcium.**

PER SERVING (about 3 cups) Calories: 317; Carbohydrates: 10g; Protein: 28g; Cholesterol: 230mg; Total Fat: 18g; Saturated Fat: 5g; Sodium: 509mg; Potassium: 546mg; Calcium: 24mg

# Egg Salad

Flare Soother | Fatigue-Friendly | Bone Booster | Gluten-Free

No-cook meals are great when you're suffering from a painful flare-up, and you can enjoy this tasty egg salad for breakfast, lunch, or dinner. While it doesn't freeze well, you can keep it in the refrigerator for up to five days, and it travels well.

**SERVES 4**
**PREP** 10 minutes
**COOK** None

¼ cup Easy Mayonnaise (page 195)

1 tablespoon Dijon mustard

½ teaspoon sea salt

⅛ teaspoon black pepper

10 large hardboiled eggs, chopped

1 cup fresh or frozen (thawed) peas

2 scallions, finely chopped

½ teaspoon smoked paprika

4 lettuce leaves

1. In a large bowl, whisk together the mayonnaise, mustard, salt, and pepper.

2. Add the eggs, peas, scallions, and paprika. Stir to combine.

3. Serve the salad scooped into the lettuce leaves.

Flare Soother Tip  Eliminate the paprika, which is a nightshade and may worsen existing inflammation in some people.

Fatigue-Friendly Tip  Buy peeled hardboiled eggs at the grocery store and chop them roughly. Eliminate the scallions.

Kidney Support Tip  Eggs are high in phosphorus, so if your doctor has suggested you watch this nutrient for your kidneys, then it's best to avoid this recipe.

Cardio Care Tip  Use 5 whole hardboiled eggs and 7 hardboiled egg whites to minimize fat and cholesterol. Reduce the salt to ¼ teaspoon to minimize sodium intake.

PER SERVING (about 1 cup) Calories: 251; Carbohydrates: 11g; Protein: 16g; Cholesterol: 413mg; Total Fat: 16g; Saturated Fat: 4g; Sodium: 540mg; Potassium: 277mg; Calcium: 48mg

# Sweet Potato Salad

Gluten-Free

Potatoes are nightshade vegetables, which can cause inflammation in some people with autoimmune disease. This version of a potato salad is made with sweet potatoes, which aren't nightshades. Leftovers will keep in the refrigerator for up to five days.

**SERVES 4**
**PREP** 10 minutes
**COOK** 15 minutes

3 sweet potatoes, peeled and cut into ¾-inch cubes

1 celery stalk, chopped

½ cup chopped yellow onion

¼ cup Easy Mayonnaise (page 195)

1 tablespoon Dijon mustard

1 tablespoon apple cider vinegar

¼ teaspoon garlic powder

½ teaspoon sea salt

⅛ teaspoon black pepper

½ teaspoon paprika

1. Put the potatoes in a large pot and add enough water to cover them. Bring the water to a boil and simmer the potatoes until soft, about 10 minutes. Drain the potatoes and allow them to cool completely.

2. In a large bowl, combine the potatoes, celery, and onion.

3. In a small bowl, whisk together the mayonnaise, mustard, vinegar, garlic powder, salt, and pepper. Add the dressing to the potatoes and toss to coat.

4. Sprinkle with the paprika and serve.

Flare Soother Tip **Eliminate the paprika, which is a nightshade and may worsen existing inflammation in some people.**

Kidney Support Tip **Replace the sweet potato, which is high in potassium, with celery root. You'll need about three celery roots. Peel and cook them just as you would the potato. Reduce the salt to ¼ teaspoon to minimize sodium intake.**

PER SERVING (about 1 cup) Calories: 295; Carbohydrates: 58g; Protein: 5g; Cholesterol: 4mg; Total Fat: 6g; Saturated Fat: <1g; Sodium: 477mg; Potassium: 1,238mg; Calcium: 24mg

# Creamy Avocado Coleslaw

Flare Soother | Fatigue-Friendly | Kidney Support | Big 8 Allergen–Free | Gluten-Free

Avocado makes a creamy dressing base for this crunchy coleslaw, which is a delicious side dish for many meals. Because avocado oxidizes quickly, it doesn't keep well, so it's best to eat this as soon as you make it. The vitamin C in the cabbage is an antioxidant that's excellent for fighting inflammation, and buying prebagged coleslaw makes this salad a snap.

**SERVES 4**
**PREP** 10 minutes
**COOK** None

1 (1-pound) bag coleslaw mix

3 scallions, chopped

½ cup Creamy Avocado Dressing (page 199)

In a large bowl, combine the coleslaw mix and scallions. Add the dressing and toss to mix. Serve.

Kidney Support Tip To lower potassium, replace the dressing with this quick recipe: Whisk together ¼ cup mayonnaise, 2 tablespoons apple cider vinegar, the juice of 1 lime, ½ teaspoon grated fresh ginger, 1 minced garlic clove, and ¼ teaspoon sea salt.

PER SERVING (about 1 cup) Calories: 134; Carbohydrates: 12g; Protein: 3g; Cholesterol: 0mg; Total Fat: 10g; Saturated Fat: 2g; Sodium: 259mg; Potassium: 468mg; Calcium: 54mg

# Ambrosia Salad

Flare Soother | Fatigue-Friendly | Kidney Support | Big 8 Allergen–Free | Gluten-Free

Coconut cream replaces the whipped topping here, making this heavenly fruit salad dairy-free and anti-inflammatory. You can buy coconut cream at some grocery stores, or you can make your own by purchasing a 14-ounce can of full-fat coconut milk and refrigerating it. Scoop the solids off the top and discard the liquid—voilà, coconut cream.

**SERVES 4**
**PREP** 10 minutes
**COOK** None

2 bananas, peeled and sliced

2 apples, peeled, cored, and sliced

1 cup blueberries

1 cup grapes, halved

1 (4-ounce) can mandarin oranges, drained

½ cup coconut cream (see headnote)

¼ cup orange juice

¼ teaspoon pure vanilla extract

1 packet stevia

1. In a large bowl, combine the bananas, apples, blueberries, grapes, and oranges.

2. In a small bowl, whisk together the coconut cream, orange juice, vanilla, and stevia.

3. Add the dressing to the fruit and toss to coat. Chill or serve immediately.

Fatigue-Friendly Tip  Buy prechopped fruit from the salad bar at the grocery store and leave the grapes whole.

Kidney Support Tip  Replace 1 banana with 1 peeled, cored, chopped pear instead.

PER SERVING (about 1 cup) Calories: 372; Carbohydrates: 43g; Protein: 2g; Cholesterol: 0mg; Total Fat: 24g; Saturated Fat: 21g; Sodium: 18mg; Potassium: 705mg; Calcium: 36mg

# Summer Berry Salad

Flare Soother | Fatigue-Friendly | Kidney Support | Cardio Care
Big 8 Allergen–Free | Gluten-Free

A simple berry salad is the perfect side dish for meat or fish. This version is super easy, because it requires little cutting or chopping. You can run the apple through a spiralizer, buy presliced apples and add them as is, or even use a vegetable peeler to peel strips of apples.

**SERVES 4**
**PREP** 10 minutes
**COOK** None

1 pint blueberries

1 pint strawberries, quartered

2 apples, spiralized
or julienned

1 tablespoon chopped
fresh mint

1 tablespoon lemon juice

1 teaspoon lemon zest

In a large bowl, combine all the ingredients and mix well. Serve.

Fatigue-Friendly Tip If you want to avoid any chopping, omit the apple and replace it with a few pints of berries that don't require any cutting or chopping, such as blackberries and raspberries. You can also purchase dried lemon zest in the spice section.

PER SERVING (about 1½ cups) Calories: 146; Carbohydrates: 37g; Protein: 2g; Cholesterol: 0mg; Total Fat: <1g; Saturated Fat: 0g; Sodium: 4mg; Potassium: 345mg; Calcium: 24mg

Baked Sweet Potato Wedges, p. 98

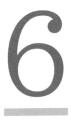

# Snacks and Sides

# Roasted Pumpkin Seeds

Flare Soother | Fatigue-Friendly | Kidney Support | Bone Booster
Big 8 Allergen–Free | Gluten-Free

Pumpkin seeds are a fabulous make-ahead snack. They'll keep in an airtight container for a few weeks, and they're packed with anti-inflammatory omega-3 fatty acids, which make them the perfect flare-up-fighting food. You can find raw pumpkin seeds at health food stores, stores like Whole Foods Market and Trader Joe's, or online.

**SERVES 8**
**PREP** 5 minutes
**COOK** 13 minutes

2 cups raw hulled pumpkin seeds

2 tablespoons extra-virgin olive oil

½ teaspoon sea salt

1. Preheat the oven to 325°F.

2. Line a baking sheet with parchment paper or aluminum foil.

3. In a medium bowl, toss the pumpkin seeds with the olive oil and salt.

4. Spread the seeds on the prepared baking sheet in a single layer. Roast until golden brown, about 13 minutes. Serve warm or cool to room temperature.

Kidney Support and Cardio Care Tip Reduce the salt to ¼ teaspoon and spice things up with 1 teaspoon ground cumin or onion powder.

PER SERVING (¼ cup) Calories: 217; Carbohydrates: 6g; Protein: 9g; Cholesterol: 0mg; Total Fat: 19g; Saturated Fat: 4g; Sodium: 123mg; Potassium: 278mg; Calcium: 12mg

# Spiced Walnuts

Flare Soother | Fatigue-Friendly | Kidney Support | Cardio Care | Bone Booster | Gluten-Free

Walnuts are a great anti-inflammatory food because of the presence of omega-3 fatty acids. These will keep for a few weeks in an airtight container, and they make a terrific on-the-go snack. They are also delicious sprinkled on salads or fruit, adding crunch and beneficial nutrients like vitamin E.

**SERVES 8**
**PREP** 5 minutes
**COOK** 10 minutes

2 cups raw walnut halves

2 tablespoons coconut oil, melted

¼ cup pure maple syrup

1 teaspoon ground cinnamon

¼ teaspoon ground allspice

¼ teaspoon ground ginger

Pinch sea salt

1. Preheat the oven to 350°F.

2. Line a baking sheet with parchment paper or aluminum foil.

3. In a medium bowl, toss the walnuts with the coconut oil, maple syrup, cinnamon, allspice, ginger, and salt.

4. Spread the nuts on the prepared baking sheet in a single layer. Roast until golden brown, 5 to 10 minutes. Serve warm or cool to room temperature.

Ingredient Tip If you're not fond of walnuts, you can use this recipe with other nuts such as pecans or almonds.

PER SERVING (¼ cup) Calories: 249; Carbohydrates: 10g; Protein: 8g; Cholesterol: 0mg; Total Fat: 22g; Saturated Fat: 4g; Sodium: 33mg; Potassium: 186mg; Calcium: 36mg

# Baked Sweet Potato Wedges

Flare Soother | Bone Booster | Big 8 Allergen–Free | Gluten-Free

Potato wedges are delicious, but they aren't always very nutritious when they are deep-fried in inflammatory industrial seed oils and sprinkled with a lot of salt. This sweet potato version is inflammation-friendly, and it has a crispy outside with a tender inside. The wedges can be delicious alone, or you can dip them in guacamole or Creamy Avocado Dressing (page 199).

**SERVES** 4
**PREP** 10 minutes
**COOK** 30 minutes

2 sweet potatoes, cut into wedges

2 tablespoons extra-virgin olive oil

1 teaspoon dried rosemary

½ teaspoon sea salt

⅛ teaspoon black pepper

1. Preheat your oven to 400°F. Line two baking sheets with parchment paper or aluminum foil.

2. In a medium bowl, toss the potatoes with the olive oil and rosemary.

3. Spread the wedges on the prepared baking sheets in a single layer. Bake for 30 minutes.

4. Sprinkle the wedges with the salt and pepper and serve warm.

Kidney Support and Cardio Care Tip Reduce the salt to ¼ teaspoon to minimize sodium intake.

PER SERVING Calories: 151; Carbohydrates: 21g; Protein: 2g; Cholesterol: 0mg; Total Fat: 7g; Saturated Fat: 1g; Sodium: 270mg; Potassium: 478mg; Calcium: 12mg

# Sesame Kale Chips

Flare Soother | Fatigue-Friendly | Kidney Support | Bone Booster
Big 8 Allergen–Free | Gluten-Free

Sesame seeds are an excellent source of calcium, and kale has plenty of anti-inflammatory nutrients that make these nutritious chips both convenient for snacking on the go and supportive of your overall health. These will keep for about a week in a tightly sealed container.

**SERVES 4**
**PREP** 10 minutes
**COOK** 15 minutes

1 bunch kale
2 tablespoons extra-virgin olive oil
½ teaspoon toasted sesame oil
2 tablespoons sesame seeds
½ teaspoon sea salt

1. Preheat the oven to 350°F.

2. Line two baking sheets with parchment paper or aluminum foil.

3. Cut away the stems and ribs from the kale leaves.

4. In a large bowl, toss the kale leaves with the olive oil, sesame oil, sesame seeds, and salt.

5. Spread the kale leaves on the prepared baking sheets in a single layer. Bake until the edges of the kale leaves brown, about 15 minutes. Serve warm.

Fatigue-Friendly Tip You can find bags of pretrimmed kale in the produce section of your grocery store. These are the perfect size to make kale chips.

Kidney Support and Cardio Care Tip Reduce the salt to ¼ teaspoon to minimize sodium and reduce the olive oil to 1 tablespoon.

PER SERVING (½ cup) Calories: 116; Carbohydrates: 6g; Protein: 2g; Cholesterol: 0mg; Total Fat: 10g; Saturated Fat: 1g; Sodium: 256mg; Potassium: 268mg; Calcium: 132mg

# Zucchini Hummus

Flare Soother | Fatigue-Friendly | Kidney Support | Big 8 Allergen–Free | Gluten-Free

Next time you want to pack a delicious, healthy snack for the office or an outing, try this variation on hummus and take along some sliced veggies. After making the hummus, you can refrigerate it for up to four days in individual serving containers. This is a great way to use zucchini when it is abundant in the late summer and early fall months.

**SERVES 4**
**PREP** 10 minutes
**COOK** None

2 zucchini, roughly chopped

1 garlic clove, minced

Juice of 1 lemon

¼ cup tahini (sesame paste)

2 tablespoons extra-virgin olive oil

½ teaspoon sea salt

1. In a blender or food processor, combine all the ingredients. Blend until smooth.

2. Serve at room temperature or chilled.

Fatigue-Friendly Tip You don't need to finely chop the zucchini here. Just give it a rough chop into 5 or 6 pieces. Use bottled lemon juice and ½ teaspoon minced garlic from a jar to save energy.

Kidney Support and Cardio Care Tip Reduce the salt to ¼ teaspoon to minimize sodium intake.

Bone Booster Tip Add calcium by replacing the zucchini with one 14-ounce can of chickpeas, rinsed and drained.

PER SERVING (¼ cup) Calories: 169; Carbohydrates: 7g; Protein: 4g; Cholesterol: 0mg; Total Fat: 15g; Saturated Fat: 2g; Sodium: 264mg; Potassium: 339mg; Calcium: 176mg

# Cauliflower Purée

Flare Soother | Fatigue-Friendly | Gluten-Free

Mashed cauliflower has become a popular side dish that many people use in place of potatoes, particularly if they are sensitive to nightshades. This version is simple and comes together quickly, but it's loaded with flavor and has a silky texture that can't be beat.

**SERVES 4**
**PREP** 10 minutes
**COOK** 10 minutes

1 head cauliflower, broken into florets

¼ cup Vegetable Broth (page 193)

¼ cup unsweetened almond milk

1 tablespoon extra-virgin olive oil

½ teaspoon onion powder

½ teaspoon sea salt

⅛ teaspoon black pepper

1. Put the cauliflower florets in a large pot and cover with water. Bring to a boil over medium-high heat and cook until the cauliflower is soft, about 10 minutes. Drain.

2. In a blender or food processor, combine the cauliflower, broth, almond milk, olive oil, onion powder, salt, and pepper. Blend until smooth. Serve warm.

Fatigue-Friendly Tip Use frozen cauliflower, or buy the cauliflower prechopped in the produce section of your grocery store.

Kidney Support and Cardio Care Tip Reduce the salt to ¼ teaspoon to minimize sodium intake.

Bone Booster Tip Add ¼ cup grated Parmesan cheese for calcium and flavor.

PER SERVING (½ cup) Calories: 53; Carbohydrates: 4g; Protein: 2g; Cholesterol: 0mg; Total Fat: 4g; Saturated Fat: <1g; Sodium: 313mg; Potassium: 229mg; Calcium: 48mg

# Cauliflower Rice

Flare Soother | Fatigue-Friendly | Kidney Support | Bone Booster
Big 8 Allergen–Free | Gluten-Free

Cauliflower rice is a delicious, nutritious, anti-inflammatory replacement for white rice, which doesn't have much to offer by way of nutrients. It's also really quick to make, particularly if you have a food processor. Use this as a base for stir-fries, or serve alongside meat dishes for a simple and flavorful side dish. You can freeze the cooked cauliflower rice in single-serving portions for up to six months.

**SERVES 4**
**PREP** 10 minutes
**COOK** 5 minutes

1 head cauliflower

2 tablespoons extra-virgin olive oil

½ teaspoon sea salt

¼ teaspoon black pepper

1. In a food processor, pulse the florets until they resemble rice. If you don't have a food processor, grate the cauliflower using the small holes of a box grater.

2. In a large sauté pan or skillet over medium-high heat, heat the olive oil until it shimmers.

3. Add the cauliflower and cook, stirring occasionally, until it softens, about 5 minutes. Season with the salt and pepper and serve.

*Kidney Support and Cardio Care Tip* **Reduce** the salt to ¼ teaspoon to minimize sodium intake.

PER SERVING (½ cup) Calories: 77; Carbohydrates: 4g; Protein: 1g; Cholesterol: 0mg; Total Fat: 7g; Saturated Fat: 1g; Sodium: 254mg; Potassium: 202mg; Calcium: 24mg

# Zucchini Noodles

Flare Soother | Fatigue-Friendly | Kidney Support | Bone Booster
Big 8 Allergen–Free | Gluten-Free

Zucchini noodles, a.k.a. "zoodles," are a great gluten-free pasta substitute. They make a tasty side dish by themselves, or you can top them with a favorite sauce or toss them in soup. The recipe includes two shape variations, so feel free to use the zoodle shape that most appeals to you.

**SERVES 4**
**PREP** 10 minutes
**COOK** 5 minutes

2 medium zucchini

2 tablespoons extra-virgin olive oil

½ teaspoon sea salt

¼ teaspoon black pepper

1. To make ribbon-style noodles, use a vegetable peeler and peel the zucchini in long, wide strips. Use as is or, to make spaghetti noodles, use a sharp knife to cut the ribbons lengthwise into thin strips.

2. In a large sauté pan or skillet over medium-high heat, heat the olive oil until it shimmers.

3. Add the zucchini and cook, stirring occasionally, until it softens, about 5 minutes. Season with the salt and pepper and serve.

Fatigue Friendly Tip If you make zoodles often, you might want to invest in a gadget called a spiralizer that allows you to cut zucchini (and other firm vegetables) into different-size noodles with little effort.

Kidney Support and Cardio Care Tip Reduce the salt to ¼ teaspoon to minimize sodium intake.

PER SERVING (½ cup) Calories: 77; Carbohydrates: 4g; Protein: 1g; Cholesterol: 0mg; Total Fat: 7g; Saturated Fat: 1g; Sodium: 254mg; Potassium: 202mg; Calcium: 24mg

# Sautéed Butternut Squash

Flare Soother | Fatigue-Friendly | Kidney Support | Bone Booster
Big 8 Allergen–Free | Gluten-Free

In this recipe, earthy butternut squash combines with sweet spices and just a hint of heat. The result is a tasty and warming side dish that complements meat, poultry, or seafood. It's a delicious way to add a little color to your meal, along with beneficial nutrients like vitamins A and C.

**SERVES 4**
**PREP** 10 minutes
**COOK** 15 minutes

2 tablespoons coconut oil
2 cups cubed
butternut squash
½ teaspoon sea salt
½ teaspoon ground cinnamon
¼ teaspoon ground ginger
¼ teaspoon ground nutmeg
Pinch ground cloves
Pinch cayenne pepper

1. In a large sauté pan or skillet over medium-high heat, heat the coconut oil until it shimmers.

2. Add the squash, salt, cinnamon, ginger, nutmeg, cloves, and cayenne.

3. Cook, stirring occasionally, until the squash is browned and soft, 10 to 15 minutes. Serve warm.

Fatigue-Friendly Tip  Buy precut fresh or frozen butternut squash at the grocery store.

Kidney Support and Cardio Care Tip  Reduce the salt to ¼ teaspoon to minimize sodium intake.

PER SERVING (½ cup)  Calories: 92; Carbohydrates: 9g; Protein: <1g; Cholesterol: 0mg; Total Fat: 7g; Saturated Fat: 6g; Sodium: 237mg; Potassium: 252mg; Calcium: 48mg

# Sweet Potato Purée

Flare Soother | Fatigue-Friendly | Kidney Support | Bone Booster | Gluten-Free

This sweet potato purée is silky and decadent. While the main recipe uses a little bit of dairy, you can adjust it (see the tips) to remove any potential allergens and make it more cardiac friendly. Experiment to discover your individual tolerances to dairy and other potentially inflammatory ingredients to minimize your chance of experiencing a flare.

**SERVES 4**
**PREP** 10 minutes
**COOK** 20 minutes

3 sweet potatoes, peeled and roughly chopped

¼ cup skim milk

2 tablespoons unsalted butter, melted

½ teaspoon sea salt

¼ teaspoon black pepper

1. Put the sweet potatoes in a large pot and cover with water. Bring to a boil over medium-high heat and cook until the potatoes are soft, 10 to 15 minutes. Drain.

2. In a blender or food processor, combine the potatoes with the milk, melted butter, salt, and pepper. Purée until smooth. Serve warm.

**Flare Soother Tip** Replace the skim milk with any unsweetened nondairy milk (but remember removing the skim milk takes away the calcium boost), and replace the butter with 1 tablespoon extra-virgin olive oil plus 1 tablespoon Vegetable Broth (page 193).

**Fatigue-Friendly Tip** Frozen sweet potato cubes will work here as well.

**Kidney Support and Cardio Care Tip** Reduce the salt to ¼ teaspoon to minimize sodium intake. Replace the butter with 2 tablespoons Vegetable Broth (page 193), and limit your consumption to a ½ cup serving.

PER SERVING (½ cup) Calories: 145; Carbohydrates: 22g; Protein: 3g; Cholesterol: 16mg; Total Fat: 6g; Saturated Fat: 4g; Sodium: 290mg; Potassium: 639mg; Calcium: 36mg

# Roasted Brussels Sprouts

Flare Soother | Fatigue-Friendly | Bone Booster | Big 8 Allergen–Free | Gluten-Free

In late fall and early winter, Brussels sprouts are abundant in grocery stores and farmers' markets. When roasted, they have an earthy, nutty flavor you'll love as a hearty side dish. They are a great source of vitamins A and C, although they are also high in potassium, so if you have kidney issues you may want to moderate your consumption of them.

**SERVES 4**
**PREP** 10 minutes
**COOK** 45 minutes

1 pound Brussels sprouts, halved lengthwise

2 tablespoons extra-virgin olive oil

½ teaspoon sea salt

¼ teaspoon black pepper

1. Preheat the oven to 400°F.

2. In a large bowl, toss the Brussels sprouts with the olive oil, salt, and pepper.

3. Spread them out, cut-side down, in a single layer on a large rimmed baking sheet.

4. Roast, stirring occasionally, until browned, 30 to 45 minutes. Serve warm.

Fatigue-Friendly Tip Whole Brussels sprouts will work here if they're small, so you don't need to halve them. The roasting time for whole Brussels sprouts will be closer to 45 minutes.

Kidney Support and Cardio Care Tip Moderation is key here. If you love Brussels sprouts, you don't need to avoid them—just cut your portion size in half. Reduce the salt to ¼ teaspoon to minimize sodium intake.

PER SERVING (1 cup) Calories: 109; Carbohydrates: 10g; Protein: 4g; Cholesterol: 0mg; Total Fat: 7g; Saturated Fat: 1g; Sodium: 262mg; Potassium: 442mg; Calcium: 48mg

# Sesame Broccoli Stir-Fry

Bone Booster | Gluten-Free

This stir-fry is delicious as a side dish or as a vegetarian main course served on a bed of Cauliflower Rice (page 102). It's also really quick and easy to prepare, requiring very little active time for a flavorful and comforting dish that's an excellent source of vitamin C and other beneficial anti-inflammatory nutrients.

**SERVES 4**
**PREP** 10 minutes
**COOK** 10 minutes

4 tablespoons extra-virgin olive oil, divided

2 cups broccoli florets

2 tablespoons gluten-free soy sauce or tamari

½ teaspoon toasted sesame oil

1 tablespoon arrowroot powder

½ teaspoon ground ginger

¼ teaspoon garlic powder

Pinch red pepper flakes (optional)

2 tablespoons sesame seeds

1. In a large sauté pan or skillet over medium-high heat, heat 2 tablespoons of olive oil until it shimmers.

2. Add the broccoli and cook, stirring occasionally, until soft, about 7 minutes.

3. In a small bowl, whisk together the soy sauce, the remaining 2 tablespoons of olive oil, sesame oil, arrowroot powder, ginger, garlic powder, and red pepper flakes (if using). Add the sauce to the pan with the broccoli.

4. Cook, stirring occasionally, until the sauce thickens, 1 to 2 minutes. Sprinkle with the sesame seeds before serving.

Flare Soother Tip Eliminate the red pepper flakes if you are sensitive to nightshades.

Kidney Support and Cardio Care Tip Reduce the soy sauce to 1 tablespoon to minimize sodium intake.

PER SERVING (½ cup) Calories: 174; Carbohydrates: 5g; Protein: 3g; Cholesterol: 0mg; Total Fat: 17g; Saturated Fat: 2g; Sodium: 467mg; Potassium: 199mg; Calcium: 154mg

# Balsamic-Glazed Mixed Vegetables

Flare Soother | Fatigue-Friendly | Kidney Support | Big 8 Allergen–Free | Gluten-Free

What could be easier than dressing up mixed veggies from the freezer section with a tasty balsamic glaze? It's a great way to make frozen vegetables more flavorful and a bit more special. You can steam the veggies in the easiest way possible—microwave or stove top—and then add them to the glaze.

**SERVES 4**
**PREP** 10 minutes
**COOK** 10 minutes

¼ cup balsamic vinegar

¼ cup honey

1 tablespoon extra-virgin olive oil

½ teaspoon onion powder

½ teaspoon ground ginger

½ teaspoon sea salt

⅛ teaspoon black pepper

2 cups frozen mixed vegetables, cooked according to package directions

1. In a large sauté pan or skillet, bring the vinegar, honey, olive oil, onion powder, ginger, salt, and pepper to a simmer over medium heat. Cook, stirring frequently, until the liquid is reduced by half, about 6 minutes.

2. Stir in the cooked vegetables to coat. Serve warm.

Kidney Support and Cardio Care Tip Reduce the salt to ¼ teaspoon to minimize sodium intake.

PER SERVING (½ cup) Calories: 158; Carbohydrates: 29g; Protein: 3g; Cholesterol: 0mg; Total Fat: 4g; Saturated Fat: <1g; Sodium: 268mg; Potassium: 179mg; Calcium: 36mg

# Honey-Glazed Carrots

Flare Soother | Fatigue-Friendly | Kidney Support | Cardio Care
Big 8 Allergen–Free | Gluten-Free

This side dish seems fancy and complicated, but it's really simple because it doesn't require any chopping. Instead, you use baby carrots, which are the perfect size for this dish but don't require any extra prep work. This showy dish is perfect to serve for company—its beautiful presentation looks like you worked hard, even when you didn't.

**SERVES 4**
**PREP** 10 minutes
**COOK** 20 minutes

1 pound baby carrots

3 tablespoons honey

1 tablespoon coconut oil

½ teaspoon ground ginger

¼ teaspoon sea salt

1. Put the carrots in a large pot and cover with water. Bring to a boil over medium-high heat and cook the carrots until soft, about 15 minutes. Drain.

2. In a sauté pan or skillet over medium heat, heat the honey and coconut oil, stirring constantly, until smooth. Add the carrots, ginger, and salt. Stir to combine and serve immediately.

Fatigue-Friendly Tip You can also use frozen carrots. Cook them according to the package directions, then toss them with the honey mixture.

PER SERVING (1 cup) Calories: 124; Carbohydrates: 24g; Protein: 1g; Cholesterol: 0mg; Total Fat: 3g; Saturated Fat: 3g; Sodium: 196mg; Potassium: 371mg; Calcium: 48mg

# Almond Meal Biscuits with Honey

Cardio Care | Gluten-Free

If you crave something from the breadbasket, try these gluten-free biscuits made with nutrient-dense almond flour in place of all-purpose flour. They are a great source of vitamin E and healthy fats. They will keep in the freezer, tightly sealed, for up to a year, so they are a great make-ahead snack.

**SERVES 12**
**PREP** 10 minutes
**COOK** 15 minutes

2½ cups almond flour

1 teaspoon baking soda

½ teaspoon sea salt

2 large eggs

2 tablespoons coconut oil, melted

2 tablespoons extra-virgin olive oil

2 tablespoons honey

1. Preheat the oven to 350°F.

2. Line a baking sheet with parchment paper or aluminum foil.

3. In a large bowl, whisk together the almond flour, baking soda, and salt.

4. In a small bowl, beat the eggs. Add the melted coconut oil, olive oil, and honey and whisk to combine.

5. Add the wet ingredients to the dry and mix until just combined.

6. Use a large spoon to scoop 12 mounds of dough onto the prepared baking sheet.

7. Bake until the biscuits are golden, about 15 minutes. Serve warm or at room temperature.

Kidney Support Tip  Reduce the salt to a pinch to minimize sodium intake.

Ingredient Tip  Almond flour is widely available in the alternative flour section of most grocery stores. If you can't find it, you can make your own by pulsing blanched almonds in a food processor until it resembles coarse sand.

PER SERVING (1 biscuit)  Calories: 175; Carbohydrates: 7g; Protein: 5g; Cholesterol: 27mg; Total Fat: 15g; Saturated Fat: 3g; Sodium: 193mg; Potassium: 157mg; Calcium: 132mg

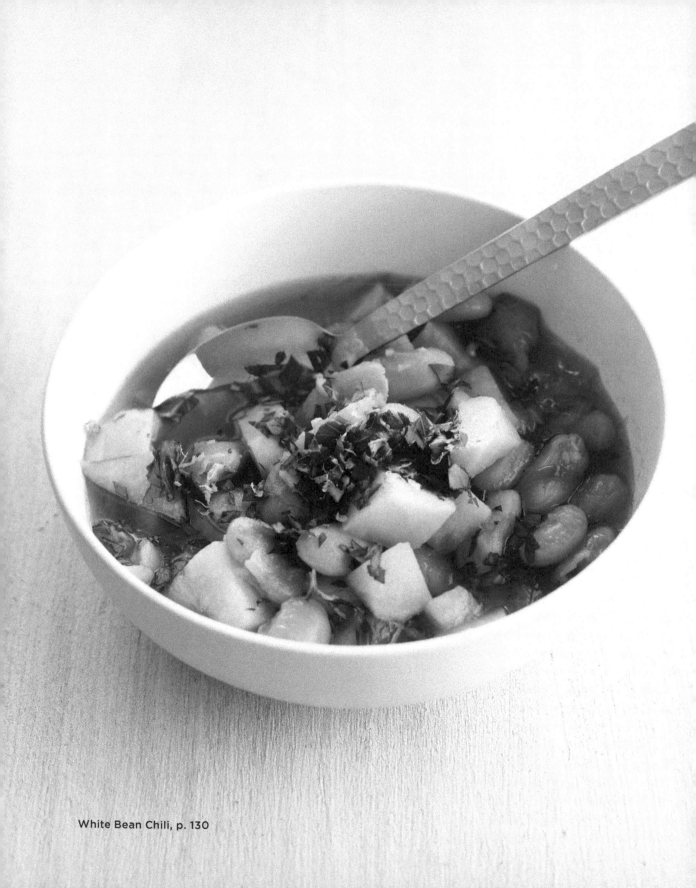

White Bean Chili, p. 130

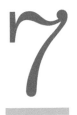

# Vegetarian and Vegan Entrées

# Veggie Pizza

Bone Booster | Gluten-Free

The crust for this delicious vegetarian pizza is made from almond and coconut flours, both of which are available in the alternative flours section of your local grocery store or online. The pesto topping is loaded with anti-inflammatory basil, walnuts, and olive oil.

**SERVES 6**
**PREP** 15 minutes
**COOK** 30 minutes

### FOR THE CRUST

Nonstick cooking spray

1 cup almond meal

½ cup coconut flour

1 teaspoon baking powder

1 teaspoon garlic powder

1 teaspoon dried oregano

4 large eggs

¼ cup extra-virgin olive oil

¼ cup almond milk

### FOR THE PESTO

¼ cup basil leaves

1 garlic clove, minced

3 tablespoons chopped walnuts

2 tablespoons extra-virgin olive oil

½ teaspoon sea salt

### TO MAKE THE CRUST

1. Preheat the oven to 375°F.

2. Coat a rimmed baking sheet or round pizza pan with nonstick cooking spray.

3. In a large bowl, whisk together the almond meal, coconut flour, baking powder, garlic powder, and oregano.

4. In another bowl, beat the eggs. Add the olive oil and almond milk and whisk to combine.

5. Add the wet ingredients to the dry and stir until it forms a batter.

6. Pour the batter onto the prepared baking sheet and spread so it is even.

7. Bake until the crust turns golden, about 15 minutes.

### TO MAKE THE PESTO

In a blender or food processor, combine all the pesto ingredients and process until well chopped.

**FOR THE TOPPINGS**

2 tablespoons extra-virgin olive oil

½ cup sliced mushrooms

½ teaspoon sea salt

1 (14-ounce) can artichoke hearts, drained

**TO MAKE THE TOPPINGS**

1. In a large sauté pan or skillet over medium-high heat, heat the olive oil until it shimmers.

2. Add the mushrooms and salt and cook, stirring occasionally, until the mushrooms are browned, about 5 minutes.

**TO MAKE THE PIZZA**

1. Spread the pesto evenly on the baked pizza crust.

2. Arrange the mushrooms and artichoke hearts on the pesto-covered pizza crust.

3. Return the pizza to the oven and bake for 10 minutes.

4. Cut into 6 slices and serve.

Kidney Support Tip Reduce the salt in the topping and pesto to ¼ teaspoon each.

Cardio Care Tip Omit the salt from the pesto. Reduce the salt in the topping to ¼ teaspoon.

PER SERVING (⅙ pizza) Calories: 393; Carbohydrates: 14g; Protein: 11g; Cholesterol: 109mg; Total Fat: 36g; Saturated Fat: 8g; Sodium: 420mg; Potassium: 587mg; Calcium: 132mg

# Asparagus Quiche

Flare Soother | Fatigue-Friendly | Kidney Support | Gluten-Free

This delightful crustless quiche keeps easily, so it's a great make-ahead meal. It will freeze in single portions for up to a year, and it reheats well in the microwave. It's perfect for lunch or dinner, particularly in spring when asparagus is in season.

**SERVES 4**
**PREP** 10 minutes
**COOK** 35 minutes

Nonstick cooking spray

2 tablespoons extra-virgin olive oil

8 ounces asparagus, trimmed

6 large eggs

½ cup unsweetened nut milk such as almond milk or lite coconut milk

1 teaspoon dried thyme

1 teaspoon onion powder

¼ teaspoon garlic powder

½ teaspoon sea salt

¼ teaspoon black pepper

1. Preheat the oven to 400°F.

2. Coat a 10-inch pie plate or a 9-inch square baking pan with nonstick cooking spray.

3. In a large sauté pan or skillet over medium-high heat, heat the olive oil until it shimmers. Add the asparagus and cook, stirring occasionally, until tender, about 5 minutes.

4. Arrange the asparagus like the spokes of a wheel in the prepared pie plate.

5. In a medium bowl, beat the eggs. Add the milk, thyme, onion powder, garlic powder, salt, and pepper and whisk to combine. Carefully pour the mixture over the asparagus.

6. Bake until the eggs are set, about 30 minutes. Cut into 4 wedges and serve.

Fatigue-Friendly Tip Replace the asparagus with 2 cups baby spinach. Cook the spinach in the olive oil just until it wilts, a minute or two, before transferring to the pie plate. Continue with the recipe as written.

Kidney Support Tip Reduce the salt to ¼ teaspoon to minimize sodium intake.

Cardio Care Tip Replace the 6 whole eggs with 6 egg whites and 2 whole eggs.

Bone Booster Tip Stir ¼ cup grated Swiss cheese into the egg mixture before adding it to the pie plate.

PER SERVING (¼ quiche) Calories: 238; Carbohydrates: 5g; Protein: 10g; Cholesterol: 246mg; Total Fat: 21g; Saturated Fat: 9g; Sodium: 333mg; Potassium: 293mg; Calcium: 72mg

# Caramelized Onion Frittata

Kidney Support | Gluten-Free

Caramelized onions add a deeply savory flavor to this simple frittata. While it takes about 40 minutes to cook, most of it is inactive time that requires you only to stir every few moments, but not much else. Leftovers will keep in the refrigerator for up to four days, and it's easy to reheat in the microwave on high for about a minute per piece.

**SERVES 4**
**PREP** 10 minutes
**COOK** 40 minutes

2 tablespoons extra-virgin olive oil

1 yellow onion, thinly sliced

1 teaspoon dried thyme

½ teaspoon sea salt

¼ teaspoon black pepper

6 large eggs

¼ cup unsweetened nut milk such as almond milk or lite coconut milk

1. In a large ovenproof sauté pan or skillet over medium-high heat, heat the olive oil until it shimmers.

2. Add the onion, thyme, salt, and pepper and cook, stirring occasionally, for 3 minutes. Reduce the heat to low and cook, stirring every few minutes, until the onions are caramelized, 20 to 25 minutes.

3. Turn on the broiler to high.

4. In a medium bowl, whisk together the eggs and milk. Carefully pour over the onions. Turn the heat to medium and cook, without stirring, until the eggs set around the edges, about 4 minutes.

5. Using a rubber spatula, pull the eggs away from the edges and tilt the pan to allow uncooked egg to flow into the spaces. Continue cooking until the eggs set again, about 2 minutes.

6. Transfer the pan to the broiler and broil until the frittata is browned and puffy, 2 to 3 minutes. Cut into 4 wedges and serve.

Fatigue-Friendly Tip You can make a large batch of caramelized onions ahead of time and freeze them in ¼-cup servings until you're ready to use them. They make a great addition to soups, stews, and other dishes.

Kidney Support and Cardio Care Tip Reduce the salt to ¼ teaspoon to minimize sodium intake. Replace the 6 whole eggs with 6 egg whites and 2 whole eggs.

Bone Booster Tip Sprinkle ¼ cup grated cheese on top of the frittata before broiling it for added calcium.

PER SERVING (¼ frittata) Calories: 201; Carbohydrates: 4g; Protein: 9g; Cholesterol: 246mg; Total Fat: 17g; Saturated Fat: 6g; Sodium: 330mg; Potassium: 172mg; Calcium: 60mg

# Spaghetti Squash Frittata

Flare Soother | Fatigue-Friendly | Kidney Support | Gluten-Free

It takes about 40 minutes to cook a spaghetti squash in your oven, but it's inactive time, and turning the squash into "spaghetti" couldn't be easier—all you have to do is scrape it with a fork. The squash is an excellent source of vitamin C and vitamin A, which are anti-inflammatory nutrients.

**SERVES 4**
**PREP** 10 minutes
**COOK** 55 minutes

½ spaghetti squash, halved lengthwise

2 tablespoons extra-virgin olive oil

½ cup chopped yellow onion

½ teaspoon dried sage

½ teaspoon sea salt

¼ teaspoon black pepper

6 large eggs

¼ cup unsweetened nut milk such as almond milk or lite coconut milk

1. Preheat the oven to 400°F.

2. Place the squash, cut-side down, on a rimmed baking sheet. Bake until it is soft, about 40 minutes.

3. Allow the squash to cool slightly. Scrape a fork across the surface to "noodle" the squash and discard the rind.

4. Turn on the broiler to high.

5. In a large ovenproof sauté pan or skillet over medium-high heat, heat the olive oil until it shimmers. Add the onion and cook, stirring occasionally, until soft, about 4 minutes.

6. Add the squash strands, sage, salt, and pepper. Cook for 2 minutes.

7. In a medium bowl, whisk together the eggs and milk. Carefully pour over the squash and onion. Turn the heat to medium and cook, without stirring, until the eggs set around the edges, about 4 minutes.

8. Using a rubber spatula, pull the eggs away from the edges and tilt the pan to allow uncooked egg to flow into the spaces. Continue cooking until the eggs set again, about 2 minutes.

9. Transfer the pan to the broiler and broil until the frittata is browned and puffy, 2 to 3 minutes. Cut into 4 wedges and serve.

**Fatigue-Friendly Tip** You can make the squash ahead of time and freeze it in ½-cup servings until you're ready to use it. Replace the chopped onion with 1 teaspoon onion powder and sauté only the squash in the olive oil for about 1 minute.

**Kidney Support and Cardio Care Tip** Reduce the salt to ¼ teaspoon to minimize sodium intake. Replace the 6 whole eggs with 6 egg whites and 2 whole eggs.

**Bone Booster Tip** Sprinkle ¼ cup grated cheese on top of the frittata before broiling it, for added calcium.

**Ingredient Tip** It can be very difficult to cut a spaghetti squash in half. To make it easier to cut, prick the squash with a fork and microwave it for 5 minutes (or roast it in the oven at 400°F for 15 minutes) to soften the squash. Then cut it in half and proceed with the recipe as written, shortening the baking time to about 30 minutes.

PER SERVING (¼ frittata) Calories: 203; Carbohydrates: 5g; Protein: 9g; Cholesterol: 246mg; Total Fat: 17g; Saturated Fat: 6g; Sodium: 334mg; Potassium: 179mg; Calcium: 60mg

# Fried Egg on a Bed of Sautéed Kale

Flare Soother | Fatigue-Friendly | Kidney Support | Cardio Care | Bone Booster | Gluten-Free

When you put an over-easy egg on top of a bed of spicy sautéed kale, the egg yolk breaks open and coats the kale, making a luxurious sauce. This is a flavorful, quick recipe that's perfect for weeknights, and it's easy to customize with your own flavor profile.

**SERVES 4**
**PREP** 10 minutes
**COOK** 15 minutes

3 tablespoons extra-virgin olive oil, divided

½ yellow onion, chopped

4 cups kale leaves, stems and ribs removed

¼ cup orange juice

½ teaspoon garlic powder

¼ teaspoon red pepper flakes

½ teaspoon sea salt, divided

4 large eggs

⅛ teaspoon black pepper

1. In a large nonstick sauté pan or skillet over medium-high heat, heat 2 tablespoons of olive oil until it shimmers.

2. Add the onion and kale and cook, stirring occasionally, for 5 minutes.

3. Add the orange juice, garlic powder, red pepper flakes, and ¼ teaspoon of salt. Cook, stirring occasionally, for 2 minutes more.

4. Remove the kale from the pan and portion onto four plates. Carefully wipe out the pan and return it to medium heat.

5. Add the remaining 1 tablespoon of olive oil to the pan, tilting the pan to spread it in an even layer on the bottom.

6. Carefully crack the eggs into the pan, making sure the whites don't run together.

7. Season the eggs with the remaining ¼ teaspoon of salt and the pepper. Cook the eggs without moving them until the whites solidify, about 4 minutes.

8. Use a spatula to carefully flip the eggs. Turn off the heat under the pan. Allow the eggs to sit in the hot pan for 1 minute more.

9. Using a spatula, carefully place the cooked eggs on the kale. Serve immediately.

Flare Soother Tip Eliminate the red pepper flakes, which are a nightshade that can increase inflammation in sensitive people.

Fatigue-Friendly Tip Buy bagged kale, which already has the ribs removed, or replace the kale with baby spinach, which requires no extra prep work. Buy prechopped onions.

PER SERVING (½ cup kale, 1 egg) Calories: 200; Carbohydrates: 11g; Protein: 8g; Cholesterol: 164mg; Total Fat: 15g; Saturated Fat: 3g; Sodium: 325mg; Potassium: 446mg; Calcium: 108mg

# Zucchini Noodles with Tri-Pepper Sauce

Kidney Support | Cardio Care | Big 8 Allergen–Free | Gluten-Free

This vegan dinner is light, fresh, and totally delicious. It uses red, orange, and yellow bell peppers to create a flavorful sauce that is delicious on its own or as a perfect pairing for proteins such as tempeh, tofu, or eggs. The sauce keeps well—in the freezer for up to a year—but it's best if you make the zucchini noodles fresh.

**SERVES 4**
**PREP** 10 minutes
**COOK** 10 minutes

2 tablespoons extra-virgin olive oil

1 red bell pepper, seeded and sliced

1 orange bell pepper, seeded and sliced

1 yellow bell pepper, seeded and sliced

1 teaspoon garlic powder

1 teaspoon onion powder

1 teaspoon dried oregano

¼ teaspoon sea salt

Pinch red pepper flakes

½ cup Vegetable Broth (page 193)

1 recipe Zucchini Noodles (page 103)

1. In a large nonstick sauté pan or skillet over medium-high heat, heat the olive oil until it shimmers.

2. Add the bell peppers, garlic powder, onion powder, oregano, salt, and red pepper flakes and cook, stirring occasionally, until the peppers are soft, about 7 minutes.

3. Add the broth and cook, stirring, for 1 minute.

4. Transfer the peppers to a blender and carefully purée until smooth, stopping to allow the steam to escape through the lid a few times as you blend.

5. Toss the sauce with the zucchini noodles and serve.

Flare Soother Tip  If you are sensitive to nightshades, it's best to avoid this recipe.

Bone Booster Tip  Toss with ¼ cup grated Parmesan or Asiago cheese before serving to boost calcium, but remember using cheese means it is no longer allergen-free.

PER SERVING (1 cup noodles, ½ cup sauce) Calories: 172; Carbohydrates: 12g; Protein: 2g; Cholesterol: 0mg; Total Fat: 15g; Saturated Fat: 3g; Sodium: 178mg; Potassium: 446mg; Calcium: 36mg

# Zucchini Noodles with Butternut Squash Sauce

Flare Soother | Fatigue-Friendly | Gluten-Free | Big 8 Allergen–Free

This earthy and flavorful vegan sauce is full of anti-inflammatory nutrients like vitamin A and vitamin C. It also makes a delicious purée or, with a little extra liquid added (about ½ cup of vegetable broth), the sauce makes a tasty soup. It keeps well in the freezer for up to a year.

**SERVES 4**
**PREP** 10 minutes
**COOK** 40 minutes

2 cups frozen butternut squash, cooked according to package directions

½ cup Vegetable Broth (page 193), hot

½ cup unsweetened nut milk, such as almond milk or lite coconut milk, heated to a simmer

1 tablespoon extra-virgin olive oil

1 teaspoon dried thyme

1 teaspoon onion powder

½ teaspoon garlic powder

½ teaspoon sea salt

¼ teaspoon black pepper

1 recipe Zucchini Noodles (page 103)

1. In a blender, combine the squash, broth, milk, olive oil, thyme, onion powder, garlic powder, salt, and pepper. Blend until smooth.

2. Toss with the zucchini noodles and serve.

Kidney Support Tip Reduce the salt to ¼ teaspoon to minimize sodium intake.

Cardio Care Tip Omit the olive oil, use almond milk instead of coconut milk, and reduce the sea salt to ¼ teaspoon to minimize sodium intake.

PER SERVING (1 cup noodles, ½ cup sauce) Calories: 220; Carbohydrates: 16g; Protein: 3g; Cholesterol: 0mg; Total Fat: 18g; Saturated Fat: 8g; Sodium: 539mg; Potassium: 724mg; Calcium: 84mg

# Stuffed Portobello Mushrooms

Flare Soother | Fatigue-Friendly | Kidney Support | Cardio Care | Gluten-Free

Spinach, artichokes, and puréed white beans make a nutritious filling for these meaty mushrooms, which are high in calcium to support your bones, while other anti-inflammatory ingredients offer nutrients like vitamin C. The vegan recipe is so simple, it's perfect for when you have a flare-up, and you can make extra and reheat them in the microwave for an easy lunch.

**SERVES 4**
**PREP** 10 minutes
**COOK** 30 minutes

2 tablespoons extra-virgin olive oil

1 yellow onion, chopped

2 cups thawed frozen spinach

1 (14-ounce) can artichoke hearts, drained

1 teaspoon garlic powder

1 teaspoon dried Italian seasoning

½ teaspoon sea salt

⅛ teaspoon black pepper

4 portobello mushroom caps, stems and gills removed

1. Preheat the oven to 350°F.

2. In a large sauté pan or skillet over medium-high heat, heat the olive oil until it shimmers. Add the onion and cook, stirring occasionally, until soft, about 5 minutes.

3. Add the spinach, artichoke hearts, garlic powder, Italian seasoning, salt, and pepper. Cook, stirring occasionally, for 3 minutes.

4. Transfer the spinach mixture to a blender or food processor and pulse until coarsely chopped.

5. Place the mushroom caps, stem-side up, on a baking sheet. Spoon the spinach mixture evenly into the mushroom caps.

6. Bake until the mushrooms are soft, about 20 minutes. Serve warm.

**Fatigue-Friendly Tip** Use 1 cup prechopped onion from the grocery store.

**Kidney Support Tip** Reduce the salt to ¼ teaspoon to minimize sodium intake.

**Bone Booster Tip** Add ½ cup grated Swiss cheese to the spinach mixture before spooning it into the mushroom caps.

PER SERVING (1 mushroom) Calories: 152; Carbohydrates: 18g; Protein: 8g; Cholesterol: 1mg; Total Fat: 8g; Saturated Fat: 1g; Sodium: 347mg; Potassium: 864mg; Calcium: 84mg

# Mushroom Stroganoff

Flare Soother | Fatigue-Friendly | Kidney Support | Gluten-Free

This quick, easy sauté features a rich sauce over hearty zucchini or sweet potato (you choose!) "noodles." The mushrooms add a deeply savory flavor that mixes beautifully with the herbs, spices, and creamy sauce in this satisfying meal. The sauce will freeze well, but you'll need to make the noodles fresh for the best results.

**SERVES 4**
**PREP** 10 minutes
**COOK** 20 minutes

2 tablespoons extra-virgin olive oil

½ yellow onion, chopped

1 pound white button or cremini mushrooms, sliced

1 teaspoon dried thyme

½ teaspoon sea salt

⅛ teaspoon black pepper

1 garlic clove, minced

1 cup unsweetened nut milk such as almond milk or lite coconut milk

1 cup Vegetable Broth (page 193)

1 tablespoon Dijon mustard

3 tablespoons arrowroot powder

3 zucchini, made into ribbons with a vegetable peeler

1. In a large sauté pan or skillet over medium-high heat, heat the olive oil until it shimmers. Add the onion and cook, stirring occasionally, until soft, about 5 minutes.

2. Add the mushrooms, thyme, salt, and pepper and cook, stirring occasionally, for 6 minutes.

3. Add the garlic and cook, stirring constantly, for 30 seconds.

4. In a small bowl, whisk together the milk, broth, mustard, and arrowroot powder. Add to the mushroom mixture. Cook, stirring constantly until it thickens, about 2 minutes.

5. Add the zucchini noodles. Cook, stirring constantly, for 3 minutes more. Serve warm.

Fatigue-Friendly Tip Use ½ teaspoon minced garlic from a jar and buy presliced mushrooms.

Kidney Support and Cardio Care Tip Reduce the salt to ¼ teaspoon to minimize sodium intake. Reduce the olive oil to 1 tablespoon to minimize fat.

Bone Booster Tip Stir in ½ cup sour cream just before serving, to boost calcium content.

PER SERVING (1 cup noodles, ½ cup sauce) Calories: 155; Carbohydrates: 19g; Protein: 6g; Cholesterol: 0mg; Total Fat: 8g; Saturated Fat: 1g; Sodium: 408mg; Potassium: 820mg; Calcium: 48mg

# Sweet Potato Curry

Flare Soother | Fatigue-Friendly | Big 8 Allergen–Free | Gluten-Free

Curry powder has a delicious flavor that complements the sweet potatoes in this recipe. It's a quick recipe that will be on your dinner table in about 30 minutes, and most of that is inactive time while the curry cooks. The curry is warming, and the sweet potatoes are nutritious and hearty.

**SERVES 4**
**PREP** 10 minutes
**COOK** 20 minutes

2 tablespoons coconut oil

1 yellow onion, chopped

1 tablespoon curry powder

3 sweet potatoes, peeled and cut into 1-inch cubes

2 cups lite coconut milk

1 cup Vegetable Broth (page 193)

1 tablespoon lime juice

½ teaspoon garlic powder

½ teaspoon sea salt

¼ cup chopped fresh cilantro

1. In a large pot over medium-high heat, heat the coconut oil until it shimmers. Add the onion and cook, stirring occasionally, until soft, about 5 minutes.

2. Add the curry powder and cook, stirring constantly, for 1 minute.

3. Add the sweet potatoes, coconut milk, broth, lime juice, garlic powder, and salt and bring to a simmer. Reduce the heat to medium and cook, stirring occasionally, until the sweet potatoes are soft, about 15 minutes. Stir in the cilantro before serving.

Fatigue-Friendly Tip Replace the sweet potatoes with 4 cups frozen butternut squash cubes and reduce the cooking time to about 7 minutes (until the squash is heated through). Use 1 cup prechopped onion.

Kidney Support Tip Reduce the salt to ¼ teaspoon to minimize sodium intake. Replace the sweet potatoes with 4 cups cubed summer squash (like zucchini or crookneck) and reduce the cooking time to about 7 minutes (until the squash is heated through).

Cardio Care Tip Replace the coconut oil with 1 tablespoon extra-virgin olive oil. Increase the broth to 2 cups and reduce the coconut milk to 1 cup.

PER SERVING (2 cups) Calories: 333; Carbohydrates: 53g; Protein: 6g; Cholesterol: 0mg; Total Fat: 13g; Saturated Fat: 12g; Sodium: 436mg; Potassium: 1,041mg; Calcium: 108mg

# White Bean Chili

Fatigue-Friendly | Bone Booster | Big 8 Allergen–Free | Gluten-Free

You can make this vegan chili easily on the stove top, or you can cook it in a slow cooker so you've got a meal ready when you get home. It's high in protein and calcium, so it's great for your bones. It also freezes really well, so you might want to make a big batch for when you'd like a quick, hearty meal. If you want a ton of flavor, include the optional green chiles in the recipe.

**SERVES 4**
**PREP** 10 minutes
**COOK** 15 minutes

2 tablespoons extra-virgin olive oil

1 yellow onion, chopped

1 cup Vegetable Broth (page 193)

2 (14-ounce) cans white beans, rinsed and drained

1 (2-ounce) can chopped green chiles (optional)

2 medium white potatoes, chopped

1 tablespoon chili powder

½ teaspoon sea salt

⅛ teaspoon black pepper

Pinch cayenne pepper

2 tablespoons chopped fresh cilantro

1. In a large pot over medium-high heat, heat the olive oil until it shimmers. Add the onion and cook, stirring occasionally, for 5 minutes.

2. Add the broth, beans, chiles with their juice (if using), potatoes, chili powder, salt, black pepper, and cayenne. Simmer, stirring occasionally, for 10 minutes. Garnish with the fresh cilantro and serve warm.

Flare Soother Tip If you are sensitive to nightshades, avoid this recipe, or replace the potatoes with 1 chopped zucchini.

Fatigue-Friendly Tip Use 1 cup prechopped onion. Omit the olive oil and combine all the remaining ingredients in a slow cooker. Cover and cook on low for 8 hours.

Kidney Support Tip This isn't a good recipe for kidney support if potassium is an issue for you. Reduce the salt to ¼ teaspoon to minimize sodium intake.

Cardio Care Tip Reduce the olive oil to 1 tablespoon and reduce the salt to ¼ teaspoon to minimize fat and sodium.

PER SERVING (2 cups) Calories: 537; Carbohydrates: 90g; Protein: 28g; Cholesterol: 0mg; Total Fat: 10g; Saturated Fat: 2g; Sodium: 480mg; Potassium: 2,609mg; Calcium: 370mg

# Red Beans and Cauliflower Rice

Fatigue-Friendly | Kidney Support | Bone Booster | Big 8 Allergen–Free | Gluten-Free

Red beans and rice are a Cajun favorite, and this vegan version is super tasty and packed with protein and calcium. The recipe also freezes and reheats well—freeze it in single-serving portions for up to a year, then reheat in the microwave for a minute or two for a quick and easy meal.

**SERVES 4**
**PREP** 10 minutes
**COOK** 10 minutes

2 tablespoons extra-virgin olive oil

1 yellow onion, chopped

1 celery stalk, chopped

1 carrot, peeled and chopped

1 green bell pepper, seeded and chopped

1 teaspoon garlic powder

1 teaspoon dried thyme

½ teaspoon dried oregano

½ teaspoon sea salt

¼ teaspoon black pepper

¼ teaspoon cayenne pepper

1 cup Vegetable Broth (page 193)

2 cups canned kidney beans, rinsed and drained

1 recipe Cauliflower Rice (page 102)

1. In a large pot over medium-high heat, heat the olive oil until it shimmers. Add the onion, celery, carrot, bell pepper, garlic powder, thyme, oregano, salt, black pepper, and cayenne and cook, stirring occasionally, for 6 minutes.

2. Add the broth and beans. Cook, stirring occasionally, until hot, about 3 minutes.

3. Stir in the cauliflower rice and serve.

Flare Soother Tip If you are sensitive to nightshades, avoid this recipe.

Fatigue-Friendly Tip Use 2 cups prechopped mirepoix (onions, celery, and carrots), which is usually available in the produce section of the grocery store.

Kidney Support Tip Minimize potassium by reducing the beans to 1 cup and eating only a half portion, along with a salad or steamed vegetables. Reduce the salt to ¼ teaspoon to minimize sodium intake.

Cardio Care Tip Reduce the olive oil to 1 tablespoon and reduce the salt to ¼ teaspoon to minimize fat and sodium.

PER SERVING (3 cups) Calories: 270; Carbohydrates: 39g; Protein: 14g; Cholesterol: 0mg; Total Fat: 8g; Saturated Fat: 1g; Sodium: 467mg; Potassium: 1,048mg; Calcium: 98mg

# Cauliflower Fried Rice

Flare Soother | Fatigue-Friendly | Cardio Care | Bone Booster | Gluten-Free

This is a great anti-inflammatory, vegetarian version of fried rice that dresses up Cauliflower Rice (page 102) with some simple flavorings and extra ingredients to give it Asian flair. This dish keeps well, so you can refrigerate it for up to four days or freeze it in individual servings for up to a year.

**SERVES 4**
**PREP** 10 minutes
**COOK** 10 minutes

2 tablespoons extra-virgin olive oil

1 bunch scallions, chopped

1 carrot, peeled and chopped

1 cup peas

2 large eggs, beaten

1 recipe Cauliflower Rice (page 102)

2 tablespoons gluten-free soy sauce or tamari

1 teaspoon ground ginger

1 teaspoon garlic powder

¼ cup chopped fresh cilantro

1. In a large sauté pan or skillet over medium-high heat, heat the olive oil until it shimmers.

2. Add the scallions, carrot, and peas and cook, stirring occasionally, until the scallions are soft, about 4 minutes.

3. Add the eggs and cook, stirring frequently, until the eggs are cooked through. Stir in the cauliflower rice.

4. Add the soy sauce, ginger, and garlic powder and cook, stirring occasionally, for 3 minutes. Stir in the cilantro before serving.

Fatigue-Friendly Tip **Replace the fresh carrots and peas with frozen carrots and peas (1½ cups total). Replace the scallions with ½ cup prechopped fresh or frozen onion.**

Kidney Support Tip **Reduce the soy sauce to 1 tablespoon or use reduced-sodium soy sauce.**

PER SERVING (1 cup) Calories: 219; Carbohydrates: 14g; Protein: 7g; Cholesterol: 82mg; Total Fat: 17g; Saturated Fat: 3g; Sodium: 518mg; Potassium: 466mg; Calcium: 72mg

# Coconut Chickpea Stew

Flare Soother | Fatigue-Friendly | Bone Booster | Big 8 Allergen–Free | Gluten-Free

Chickpeas are an excellent source of calcium and protein, while the other veggies add nutrients like vitamin C, vitamin A, and vitamin E, which are all excellent for inflammation. Serve this stew atop Cauliflower Rice (page 102) for a hearty, flavorful meal.

**SERVES 4**
**PREP** 5 minutes
**COOK** 12 minutes

2 tablespoons extra-virgin olive oil

1 yellow onion, chopped

2 cups frozen peas and carrots

2 (14-ounce) cans chickpeas, rinsed and drained

1 cup Vegetable Broth (page 193)

1 cup lite coconut milk

¼ cup orange juice

1 teaspoon garlic powder

1 teaspoon ground ginger

¼ teaspoon ground nutmeg

½ teaspoon sea salt

⅛ teaspoon black pepper

1. In a large pot over medium-high heat, heat the olive oil until it shimmers. Add the onion and cook, stirring occasionally, for 6 minutes.

2. Add the peas and carrots, chickpeas, broth, coconut milk, orange juice, garlic powder, ginger, nutmeg, salt, and pepper and bring to a simmer. Cook, stirring, for 5 minutes. Serve warm.

Fatigue-Friendly Tip Use 1 cup prechopped onion.

Kidney Support Tip Reduce your portion size by half to minimize potassium, and serve with a side of salad or steamed vegetables. Reduce the salt to ¼ teaspoon to minimize sodium intake.

Cardio Care Tip Reduce the olive oil to 1 tablespoon and reduce the salt to ¼ teaspoon to minimize fat and sodium.

PER SERVING (2 cups) Calories: 438; Carbohydrates: 61g; Protein: 20g; Cholesterol: 0mg; Total Fat: 15g; Saturated Fat: 5g; Sodium: 514mg; Potassium: 922mg; Calcium: 132mg

# Mexican Black Bean Stew

Flare Soother | Fatigue-Friendly | Kidney Support | Big 8 Allergen–Free | Gluten-Free

You can make this stew on the stove top, or just place all the ingredients (minus the olive oil) in a slow cooker and set it on low to cook all day (6 to 8 hours) so you have a meal ready when you get home. It's a tasty and hearty vegan meal that's packed with protein and flavor—the perfect combination.

**SERVES 4**
**PREP** 5 minutes
**COOK** 18 minutes

2 tablespoons extra-virgin olive oil

1 yellow onion, chopped

1 garlic clove, minced

1 cup Vegetable Broth (page 193)

2 (14-ounce) cans black beans, rinsed and drained

1 (2-ounce) can chopped green chiles

3 cups frozen chopped carrots

Grated zest and juice of 1 lime

1 teaspoon onion powder

1 teaspoon chili powder

1 teaspoon ground cumin

½ teaspoon ground coriander

½ teaspoon sea salt

Pinch cayenne pepper

1. In a large pot over medium-high heat, heat the olive oil until it shimmers. Add the onion and cook, stirring occasionally, for 6 minutes. Add the garlic and cook, stirring constantly, for 30 seconds.

2. Add the broth, beans, chiles with their juice, carrots, lime zest and juice, onion powder, chili powder, cumin, coriander, salt, and cayenne.

3. Simmer, stirring occasionally, for 10 minutes. Serve warm.

**Flare Soother Tip** Omit the green chiles and the chili powder, both of which are nightshades.

- - - - - - - - - - - - - - - - - - - - - - - - - - - - - -

**Fatigue-Friendly Tip** Use ½ teaspoon minced garlic from a jar and prechopped onion.

- - - - - - - - - - - - - - - - - - - - - - - - - - - - - -

**Kidney Support Tip** Reduce your portion by half to minimize potassium, and serve with a salad or side of Cauliflower Rice (page 102). Avoid high-potassium foods for the rest of the day. Reduce the salt to ¼ teaspoon to minimize sodium intake.

- - - - - - - - - - - - - - - - - - - - - - - - - - - - - -

**Cardio Care Tip** Reduce the olive oil to 1 tablespoon and reduce the salt to ¼ teaspoon to minimize fat and sodium.

- - - - - - - - - - - - - - - - - - - - - - - - - - - - - -

**Bone Booster Tip** Serve each portion with 2 tablespoons sour cream and ¼ cup grated Monterey Jack cheese to boost calcium, but remember using dairy means it is no longer allergen-free.

PER SERVING (2 cups) Calories: 498; Carbohydrates: 85g; Protein: 24g; Cholesterol: 0mg; Total Fat: 9g; Saturated Fat: 2g; Sodium: 415mg; Potassium: 2,058mg; Calcium: 216mg

Cod and Chickpea Packets, p. 143

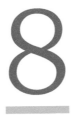

# Seafood Entrées

# Easy Tuna Casserole

Flare Soother | Fatigue-Friendly | Kidney Support | Gluten-Free

Tuna, mushrooms, peas, and sweet potato "noodles" offer a nutritious alternative to the traditional tuna noodle casserole. Dried mushrooms and broth create the flavorful gravy. The result is a flavorful and hearty casserole that makes a great family meal.

**SERVES 4**
**PREP** 10 minutes
(plus 2 hours inactive)
**COOK** 1 hour

2 ounces dried mushrooms

3 cups Chicken Broth (page 192)

1 tablespoon extra-virgin olive oil

1 yellow onion, chopped

1 cup sliced mushrooms

1 cup peas

1 garlic clove, minced

1 teaspoon dried thyme

3 tablespoons arrowroot powder

1 sweet potato, peeled and made into ribbons with a vegetable peeler

2 (5-ounce) cans water-packed tuna, drained

½ teaspoon sea salt

⅛ teaspoon black pepper

1. In a medium saucepan, bring the mushrooms and broth to a boil. Turn off the heat and cover. Allow the mushrooms to steep and flavor the broth for 2 hours. Strain the mushrooms from the broth and discard them.

2. Preheat the oven to 350°F.

3. In a large nonstick sauté pan or skillet over medium-high heat, heat the olive oil until it shimmers.

4. Add the onion, mushrooms, and peas. Cook, stirring occasionally, until the veggies are soft, about 5 minutes.

5. Add the garlic and thyme and cook, stirring constantly, for 30 seconds.

6. Whisk the arrowroot powder into the mushroom-flavored broth. Stir it into the pan with the veggies. Cook, stirring occasionally, until the broth thickens, about 30 minutes.

7. Stir in the sweet potato noodles, tuna, salt, and pepper.

8. Transfer the mixture to a 9-inch square baking pan. Bake until bubbly, 25 to 30 minutes. Serve warm.

Fatigue-Friendly Tip  Use ½ teaspoon minced garlic from a jar, and buy presliced mushrooms. Use any type of veggie noodles you can find already prepared in the grocery store produce section.

Kidney Support and Cardio Care Tip  Reduce the salt to ¼ teaspoon to minimize sodium intake. Use low-sodium tuna.

PER SERVING (1 cup)  Calories: 249; Carbohydrates: 16g; Protein: 24g; Cholesterol: 22mg; Total Fat: 10g; Saturated Fat: 2g; Sodium: 338mg; Potassium: 589mg; Calcium: 36mg

# Tuna Melt

Flare Soother | Fatigue-Friendly | Kidney Support | Bone Booster | Gluten-Free

Instead of using bread for a tuna sandwich, how about making an open-faced mushroom stuffed with tuna salad with a little cheese melted over the top? The cheese is a bone-building addition to this healthy dish.

**SERVES 4**
**PREP** 10 minutes
**COOK** 25 minutes

1½ cups water-packed tuna, drained

½ cup peas

3 scallions, chopped

¼ cup Easy Mayonnaise (page 195)

2 tablespoons Dijon mustard

1 teaspoon dried tarragon

¼ teaspoon sea salt

4 portobello mushroom caps, stems and gills removed

4 ounces low-fat cheddar cheese, grated

1. Preheat the oven to 425°F.

2. In a medium bowl, mix the tuna, peas, scallions, mayonnaise, mustard, tarragon, and salt.

3. Place the mushroom caps on a rimmed baking sheet, stem-side up, and fill with the tuna mixture.

4. Top with the cheese.

5. Bake until the mushrooms are soft and the cheese is melted and bubbly, about 25 minutes. Serve warm.

Fatigue-Friendly Tip Omit the scallions. Buy pregrated cheese, or omit it.

Kidney Support and Cardio Care Tip Omit the salt to reduce sodium.

PER SERVING (½ cup tuna salad, 1 portobello mushroom) Calories: 379; Carbohydrates: 11g; Protein: 35g; Cholesterol: 61mg; Total Fat: 22g; Saturated Fat: 8g; Sodium: 538mg; Potassium: 687mg; Calcium: 300mg

# Fish and Chips

Flare Soother | Fatigue-Friendly | Bone Booster | Gluten-Free

Fish and chips is a popular entrée that many people enjoy, but it tends to be high in fat and inflammatory ingredients. This recipe omits inflammatory ingredients like bread crumbs and industrial seed oils and contains plenty of healthy fats to fight inflammation.

**SERVES 4**
**PREP** 10 minutes
**COOK** 20 minutes

1 large egg plus 1 large egg white

¼ cup almond milk

2 tablespoons Dijon mustard

1 cup almond meal

1 teaspoon dried thyme

1 teaspoon onion powder

¼ teaspoon sea salt

¼ teaspoon black pepper

12 ounces cod, cut into four pieces

1 recipe Baked Sweet Potato Wedges (page 98)

1. Preheat the oven to 425°F.

2. In a medium bowl, whisk together the egg, egg white, almond milk, and mustard.

3. In another bowl, mix the almond meal, thyme, onion powder, salt, and pepper.

4. Dredge the fish in the egg mixture and then in the almond meal mixture, tapping off any excess.

5. Place the coated fish on a rimmed baking sheet. Bake until cooked through, about 20 minutes. Serve with the sweet potato wedges.

Kidney Support Tip  Replace the sweet potato wedges with a side salad to reduce potassium.

Cardio Care Tip  Use 3 egg whites in place of the whole egg to reduce cholesterol and fat.

PER SERVING (3 ounces cod) Calories: 411; Carbohydrates: 29g; Protein: 28g; Cholesterol: 88mg; Total Fat: 21g; Saturated Fat: 3g; Sodium: 426mg; Potassium: 1046mg; Calcium: 132mg

# Lemon Pepper Cod

Flare Soother | Fatigue-Friendly | Kidney Support | Gluten-Free

This is a super easy main course. Serve it alongside a simple salad or any of the veggie side dish recipes in chapter 6 (such as the Roasted Brussels Sprouts on page 106) for a delicious and satisfying meal your whole family will love. While freshly squeezed lemon juice tastes better than the stuff that comes in a bottle, if you're experiencing a flare-up, by all means go for the convenience of the bottled lemon juice.

**SERVES 4**
**PREP** 10 minutes
**COOK** 10 minutes

2 tablespoons extra-virgin olive oil

12 ounces cod, cut into four pieces

¼ teaspoon sea salt

½ teaspoon black pepper

¼ cup lemon juice

1. In a large nonstick sauté pan or skillet over medium-high heat, heat the olive oil until it shimmers.

2. Sprinkle the cod on both sides with the salt and pepper.

3. Add the cod to the pan and cook, flipping once, until opaque and flaky, about 5 minutes per side. Sprinkle both sides with the lemon juice as it cooks. Serve immediately.

Cardio Care Tip  Reduce the olive oil to 1 tablespoon.

PER SERVING (3 ounces cod) Calories: 154; Carbohydrates: <1g; Protein: 20g; Cholesterol: 47mg; Total Fat: 8g; Saturated Fat: 1g; Sodium: 187mg; Potassium: 230mg; Calcium: 12mg

# Cod and Chickpea Packets

Flare Soother | Gluten-Free

For this no-fuss, no-mess meal, earthy chickpeas and cod are delicately flavored with thyme and lemon. Because all of it is wrapped up in a foil or parchment packet and baked in the oven, it's perfect for when you're not feeling like spending a long time in the kitchen.

**SERVES 4**
**PREP** 10 minutes
**COOK** 20 minutes

1 (15-ounce) can chickpeas, drained

1 zucchini, thinly sliced lengthwise with a vegetable peeler

4 thyme sprigs

16 cherry tomatoes

12 ounces cod, cut into four pieces

1 tablespoon extra-virgin olive oil

½ teaspoon sea salt

¼ teaspoon black pepper

½ cup lemon juice

1. Preheat the oven to 400°F.

2. Fold four large squares of aluminum foil into packets, leaving room to fold the opening closed. Place the packets on a rimmed baking sheet.

3. Place the chickpeas, zucchini, thyme, and tomatoes in the packets. Top with the cod. Drizzle the cod with the olive oil and then sprinkle with the salt and pepper.

4. Carefully pour the orange juice around the edges of the cod.

5. Seal the foil at the opening to make closed packets and bake until the cod is opaque and flaky, 15 to 20 minutes.

6. Serve in the packets to minimize cleanup.

Kidney Support and Cardio Care Tip Reduce the salt to ¼ teaspoon to minimize sodium intake. Replace the chickpeas with green peas (2 cups) to reduce potassium.

Flare Soother Tip Omit the cherry tomatoes if you are sensitive to nightshades.

PER SERVING Calories: 610; Carbohydrates: 86g; Protein: 45g; Cholesterol: 47mg; Total Fat: 12g; Saturated Fat: 2g; Sodium: 361mg; Potassium: 2,472mg; Calcium: 36mg

# Asian Salmon with Spicy Coleslaw

Flare Soother | Fatigue-Friendly | Kidney Support | Cardio Care | Bone Booster | Gluten-Free

This dish is a feast for your senses, with crunchy, spicy coleslaw and rich, flavorful marinated salmon. It's also a quick and easy dinner you can have on the table in 30 minutes, and it contains nutritious, anti-inflammatory ingredients like omega-3 fatty acids, ginger, and vitamin C.

**SERVES 4**
**PREP** 20 minutes (10 inactive)
**COOK** 10 minutes

### FOR THE SALMON

¼ cup rice vinegar

2 tablespoons lime juice

2 tablespoons honey

1 tablespoon gluten-free soy sauce or tamari

2 teaspoons ground ginger

½ teaspoon garlic powder

⅛ teaspoon cayenne pepper

12 ounces salmon, cut into four pieces

1 tablespoon extra-virgin olive oil

### TO MAKE THE SALMON

1. In a small bowl, whisk together the rice vinegar, lime juice, honey, soy sauce, ginger, garlic powder, and cayenne. Pour into a small baking dish or pie plate.

2. Place the salmon in the mixture, flesh-side down, and marinate for 10 minutes.

3. In a large sauté pan over medium-high heat, heat the olive oil until it shimmers.

4. Remove the salmon from the marinade and pat it dry.

5. Add the salmon to the pan and cook, flipping once, until opaque and flaky, about 4 minutes per side.

**FOR THE COLESLAW**

2 cups coleslaw mix

2 tablespoons apple cider vinegar

2 tablespoons extra-virgin olive oil

1 tablespoon lime juice

1 teaspoon honey

⅛ teaspoon sriracha

1 garlic clove, minced

1 teaspoon ground ginger

**TO MAKE THE COLESLAW**

1. Put the coleslaw mix in a medium bowl.

2. In a small bowl, whisk together the vinegar, olive oil, lime juice, honey, sriracha, garlic, and ginger.

3. Toss the dressing with the coleslaw.

4. Serve the salmon on top of the coleslaw.

Flare Soother Tip Eliminate the cayenne and sriracha if nightshades are an issue for you.

Fatigue-Friendly Tip Use ½ teaspoon minced garlic from a jar.

PER SERVING (3 ounces salmon, ½ cup coleslaw) Calories: 272; Carbohydrates: 14g; Protein: 18g; Cholesterol: 38mg; Total Fat: 16g; Saturated Fat: 2g; Sodium: 274mg; Potassium: 445mg; Calcium: 60mg

# Orange-Honey Glazed Salmon

Flare Soother | Fatigue-Friendly | Kidney Support | Cardio Care | Gluten-Free

Salmon is packed with inflammation-soothing omega-3 fatty acids. While this makes salmon a bit higher in fat than other fish, it's the good kind of fat that supports your body by reducing inflammation and providing a great source of vitamin E. Serve this with a simple salad or alongside steamed asparagus for a complete and filling meal.

**SERVES 4**
**PREP** 10 minutes
**COOK** 13 minutes

½ cup orange juice

¼ cup honey

1 tablespoon gluten-free soy sauce or tamari

12 ounces salmon, cut into four pieces

2 tablespoons extra-virgin olive oil

¼ teaspoon black pepper

1. In a small bowl, whisk together the orange juice, honey, and soy sauce. Pour into a small baking dish or pie plate.

2. Place the salmon in the mixture, flesh-side down, and marinate for 10 minutes.

3. In a large, nonstick sauté pan or skillet over medium-high heat, heat the olive oil until it shimmers.

4. Remove the salmon from the marinade and pat it dry with a paper towel. Sprinkle it with the pepper.

5. Add the salmon to the pan, flesh-side down, and cook for 4 minutes. Flip and continue cooking until the salmon is opaque, 3 to 4 minutes more.

6. While the salmon cooks, bring the marinade to a boil in a small saucepan. Boil for 4 minutes.

7. Spoon the cooked marinade over the salmon and serve.

Ingredient Tip Before you marinate the salmon, use a pair of needle-nose pliers to remove the small pin bones from the fish.

PER SERVING (3 ounces salmon) Calories: 253; Carbohydrates: 21g; Protein: 17g; Cholesterol: 38mg; Total Fat: 12g; Saturated Fat: 2g; Sodium: 264mg; Potassium: 410mg; Calcium: 36mg

# Salmon and Summer Squash

Flare Soother | Fatigue-Friendly | Kidney Support | Gluten-Free

Cooking fish in foil packets not only ensures that the salmon is nice and moist, but it also minimizes cleanup time, because all you need to do is throw away the packets. While the cooking method suggests using your oven, you can also cook these packets on an outdoor grill over indirect heat.

**SERVES 4**
**PREP** 10 minutes
**COOK** 20 minutes

1 medium yellow squash, sliced

1 medium zucchini, sliced

½ cup chopped yellow onion

12 ounces salmon, cut into four pieces

1 teaspoon dried thyme

½ teaspoon sea salt

⅛ teaspoon black pepper

¼ cup lemon juice

1. Preheat the oven to 400°F.

2. Fold four large squares of aluminum foil into packets, leaving room to fold the opening closed. Place the packets on a rimmed baking sheet.

3. Divide the squash, zucchini, and onion evenly among the packets.

4. Place a piece of salmon on top. Sprinkle with the thyme, salt, and pepper. Sprinkle with the lemon juice.

5. Seal the foil at the opening to make closed packets and bake until the salmon is opaque, about 20 minutes.

6. Serve in the packets to minimize cleanup.

Fatigue-Friendly Tip Use a mandoline or the slicer attachment on a food processor to slice the squash and zucchini. Use pre-chopped onion.

Kidney Support and Cardio Care Tip Reduce the salt to ¼ teaspoon to minimize sodium intake.

PER SERVING (3 ounces salmon, ½ cup squash) Calories: 138; Carbohydrates: 5g; Protein: 18g; Cholesterol: 38mg; Total Fat: 6g; Saturated Fat: <1g; Sodium: 385mg; Potassium: 626mg; Calcium: 60mg

# Baked White Fish with Mango Salsa

Flare Soother | Fatigue-Friendly | Kidney Support | Cardio Care | Gluten-Free

You can use any affordable white fish readily available in your grocery store, such as halibut, snapper, or cod. This recipe is high in vitamin A and vitamin E, which makes it a great flare soother. Serve it with a side of Cauliflower Rice (page 102) for a nutritious meal.

**SERVES 4**
**PREP** 20 minutes
**COOK** 20 minutes

12 ounces white fish, cut into four pieces

¼ teaspoon sea salt, divided

¼ teaspoon black pepper

1 cup cubed mango

½ cup chopped red onion

1 tablespoon lime juice

2 tablespoons chopped fresh cilantro

1. Preheat the oven to 350°F.

2. Season the fish with ⅛ teaspoon of salt and the pepper. Place it on a baking sheet.

3. Bake until the fish is opaque, 15 to 20 minutes.

4. In a small bowl, combine the mango, onion, lime juice, cilantro, and remaining ⅛ teaspoon of salt.

5. Top the cooked fish with the salsa and serve.

Fatigue-Friendly Tip **Use frozen (thawed) cubed mango, prechopped red onion, and freeze-dried chopped cilantro.**

PER SERVING (3 ounces fish, ¼ cup salsa) Calories: 147; Carbohydrates: 14g; Protein: 20g; Cholesterol: 47mg; Total Fat: 1g; Saturated Fat: 0g; Sodium: 186mg; Potassium: 378mg; Calcium: 24mg

# White Fish with Cranberry Compote

Flare Soother | Fatigue-Friendly | Gluten-Free

The fresh cranberries add lots of flavor to this compote, which serves as a sauce for the fish. Use any mild white fish you like, such as halibut, snapper, or cod. Serve alongside a simple tossed salad or any of the veggie side dishes in chapter 6 for a balanced and nutritious meal.

**SERVES 4**
**PREP** 10 minutes
**COOK** 15 minutes

12 ounces white fish, cut into four pieces

½ teaspoon sea salt

¼ teaspoon black pepper

1 tablespoon extra-virgin olive oil

½ cup orange juice

2 cups fresh cranberries

1 teaspoon ground ginger

1. Season the fish with the salt and pepper.

2. In a large, nonstick sauté pan or skillet over medium-high heat, heat the olive oil until it shimmers.

3. Add the fish and cook, flipping once, until opaque, about 4 minutes per side.

4. Transfer the fish to a platter and tent with aluminum foil to keep warm.

5. Add the orange juice, cranberries, and ginger to the same pan. Cook, stirring occasionally, until the cranberries start to pop, about 7 minutes.

6. Spoon the compote over the fish and serve.

Kidney Support and Cardio Care Tip Reduce the salt to ¼ teaspoon to minimize sodium intake.

PER SERVING (3 ounces fish, ¼ cup compote) Calories: 165; Carbohydrates: 9g; Protein: 20g; Cholesterol: 47mg; Total Fat: 4g; Saturated Fat: <1g; Sodium: 184mg; Potassium: 371mg; Calcium: 24mg

# White Fish Cakes with Lemon-Lime Aioli

Kidney Support | Bone Booster | Gluten-Free

White fish flakes really well when you run a fork over it, making it perfect for these simple and flavorful fish cakes. Instead of using bread crumbs to bind the cakes, use a little almond meal, which adds healthy fats and vitamin E to the cakes. Serve with a salad or a side of steamed veggies.

**SERVES 4**
**PREP** 10 minutes
**COOK** 30 minutes

**FOR THE FISH CAKES**

12 ounces white fish, cooked and flaked

¼ cup almond meal

2 tablespoons Easy Mayonnaise (page 195)

1 tablespoon Dijon mustard

1 teaspoon dried tarragon

1 teaspoon dried thyme

1 teaspoon onion powder

½ teaspoon garlic powder

¼ teaspoon sea salt

⅛ teaspoon black pepper

**FOR THE AIOLI**

½ cup Easy Mayonnaise (page 195)

½ teaspoon grated lime zest

½ teaspoon grated lemon zest

**TO MAKE THE FISH CAKES**

1. Preheat the oven to 375°F.

2. Line a baking sheet with parchment paper or aluminum foil.

3. In a medium bowl, combine the fish and almond meal.

4. In another bowl, whisk together the mayonnaise, mustard, tarragon, thyme, onion powder, garlic powder, salt, and pepper.

5. Mix the dressing with the fish. Form into 8 cakes and place on the prepared baking sheet.

6. Bake for 15 minutes. Flip and bake for an additional 15 minutes.

**TO MAKE THE AIOLI**

1. In a small bowl, whisk together the mayonnaise and the lemon and lime zest.

2. Spoon the aioli on top of the fish cakes and serve.

Flare Soother Tip **Replace the mayonnaise with an equal amount of plain yogurt if you aren't sensitive to dairy but are sensitive to eggs.**

Kidney Support and Cardio Care Tip **Reduce the salt to ¼ teaspoon to minimize sodium intake.**

PER SERVING (2 fish cakes, 2 tablespoons aioli) Calories: 274; Carbohydrates: 11g; Protein: 21g; Cholesterol: 56mg; Total Fat: 16g; Saturated Fat: 2g; Sodium: 490mg; Potassium: 277mg; Calcium: 48mg

# White Fish and Stone Fruit Packets

Flare Soother | Fatigue-Friendly | Kidney Support | Gluten-Free

Light fish and slightly sweet fruit combine in this tasty meal. Serve with a salad or a side of steamed veggies for a nutritious dinner that takes little effort to prepare or clean up. Cooking in a foil packet keeps the fish moist and allows the fruits to soften as they cook.

**SERVES 4**
**PREP** 10 minutes
**COOK** 20 minutes

12 ounces white fish, cut into four pieces

1 teaspoon dried thyme

½ teaspoon sea salt

⅛ teaspoon black pepper

2 peaches, peeled, pitted, and chopped

2 plums, peeled, pitted, and chopped

1. Preheat the oven to 400°F.

2. Fold four large squares of aluminum foil into packets, leaving room to fold the opening closed. Place the packets on a baking sheet.

3. Place one fish piece in each packet. Sprinkle with the thyme, salt, and pepper.

4. Arrange the chopped peaches and plums on top of the fish.

5. Seal the foil closed at the top to make closed packets and bake until the fish is opaque and flaky, 15 to 20 minutes.

6. Serve in the packets to minimize cleanup.

Fatigue-Friendly Tip Use frozen chopped peaches (2 cups) and omit the plums.

Kidney Support and Cardio Care Tip Reduce the salt to ¼ teaspoon to minimize sodium intake.

PER SERVING (3 ounces fish, ¼ cup fruit) Calories: 135; Carbohydrates: 11g; Protein: 20g; Cholesterol: 47mg; Total Fat: 1g; Saturated Fat: 0g; Sodium: 301mg; Potassium: 405mg; Calcium: 24mg

# Coconut Fish Curry

Flare Soother | Fatigue-Friendly | Kidney Support | Bone Booster | Gluten-Free

Ginger and turmeric can help keep inflammation at bay while adding tremendous flavor to this fish curry. It cooks on the stove top in about 20 minutes, so it's as quick to make as it is tasty. Serve the curry with Cauliflower Rice (page 102) stirred right in for an even heartier meal.

**SERVES 4**
**PREP** 10 minutes
**COOK** 25 minutes

1 tablespoon coconut oil

1 yellow onion, chopped

1 carrot, peeled and chopped

1 teaspoon curry powder

3 cups Chicken Broth (page 192)

1 cup lite coconut milk

1 sweet potato, peeled and cubed

½ teaspoon ground ginger

½ teaspoon ground turmeric

½ teaspoon garlic powder

½ teaspoon sea salt

12 ounces white fish, cut into bite-size pieces

1 tablespoon lime juice

2 tablespoons chopped fresh cilantro

1. In a large pot over medium-high heat, heat the coconut oil until it shimmers.

2. Add the onion, carrot, and curry powder. Cook, stirring occasionally, for 5 minutes.

3. Add the broth, coconut milk, sweet potato, ginger, turmeric, garlic powder, and salt. Cook, stirring occasionally, until the potatoes soften, about 15 minutes.

4. Add the fish and continue cooking until the fish is cooked through, about 5 minutes more. Sprinkle with the lime juice and cilantro and serve.

Fatigue-Friendly Tip **Use frozen (thawed) chopped carrots and prechopped onions.**

Kidney Support Tip **Omit the chopped carrots and replace the sweet potato with 1½ cups baby carrots to reduce potassium.**

Cardio Care Tip **Reduce the salt to ¼ teaspoon to minimize sodium intake. Replace the coconut oil with olive oil to reduce saturated fat.**

PER SERVING (2 cups) Calories: 230; Carbohydrates: 14g; Protein: 25g; Cholesterol: 47mg; Total Fat: 8g; Saturated Fat: 6g; Sodium: 911mg; Potassium: 617mg; Calcium: 48mg

# Trout with Green Beans and Almonds

Flare Soother | Fatigue-Friendly | Kidney Support | Cardio Care | Bone Booster | Gluten-Free

Almonds are a great source of vitamin E, while trout is a nutritious source of omega-3 fatty acids and protein. Together they make a great anti-inflammatory meal. Cooking the fish in the oven in foil packets also means it's a super easy meal to prepare when you're in the middle of a flare-up.

**SERVES 4**
**PREP** 20 minutes
**COOK** 20 minutes

2 cups frozen green beans

¼ cup slivered almonds

1 pound trout, skin on, cut into four pieces

1 tablespoon extra-virgin olive oil

½ teaspoon dried tarragon

¼ teaspoon sea salt

¼ teaspoon black pepper

¼ cup orange juice

1. Preheat the oven to 400°F.

2. Fold four large squares of aluminum foil into packets, leaving room to fold the opening closed. Place the packets on a rimmed baking sheet.

3. Divide the green beans and almonds among the packets, then top with the trout, skin-side down.

4. Brush the trout with the olive oil and sprinkle it with the tarragon, salt, and pepper.

5. Carefully pour the orange juice around the edges of the trout.

6. Seal the foil at the opening to make closed packets and bake until the fish is opaque, 15 to 20 minutes. Remove the skin before serving.

7. Serve in the packets to minimize cleanup.

Ingredient Tip Place the trout in good light, skin-side down, so you can see any pin bones. Remove the bones with needle-nose pliers before adding the fish to the foil packets.

PER SERVING (4 ounces trout, ½ cup beans) Calories: 304; Carbohydrates: 7g; Protein: 32g; Cholesterol: 84mg; Total Fat: 16g; Saturated Fat: 2g; Sodium: 197mg; Potassium: 719mg; Calcium: 120mg

# Shrimp Scampi on Zucchini Noodles

Flare Soother | Fatigue-Friendly | Kidney Support | Gluten-Free

Serve this easy main course over a bed of zucchini noodles for a wholesome meal. To save time, buy frozen shelled, deveined shrimp. Thaw them in a colander in the sink under running water, which takes about 10 minutes.

**SERVES 4**
**PREP** 10 minutes
**COOK** 7 minutes

2 tablespoons extra-virgin olive oil

12 ounces peeled, deveined shrimp

1 teaspoon dried Italian seasoning

2 garlic cloves, minced

¼ cup lemon juice

¼ teaspoon sea salt

⅛ teaspoon black pepper

Pinch red pepper flakes

1 recipe Zucchini Noodles (page 103)

1. In a large, nonstick sauté pan or skillet over medium-high heat, heat the olive oil until it shimmers.

2. Add the shrimp and Italian seasoning. Cook, stirring frequently, until the shrimp are pink and opaque, about 5 minutes.

3. Add the garlic and cook, stirring constantly, for 30 seconds.

4. Add the lemon juice, salt, black pepper, and red pepper flakes. Cook for 1 minute more to allow the flavors to blend.

5. Spoon the shrimp scampi over the zucchini noodles and serve.

Flare Soother Tip Omit the red pepper flakes if you are sensitive to nightshades. You can also add a tablespoon of chopped fresh parsley to give the dish an anti-inflammatory boost.

Fatigue-Friendly Tip Use ½ teaspoon minced garlic from a jar.

Cardio Care Tip Reduce the olive oil to 1 tablespoon.

Bone Booster Tip Sprinkle each portion with 2 tablespoons grated Parmesan or Asiago cheese to boost calcium.

PER SERVING (3 ounces shrimp, ½ cup zucchini noodles) Calories: 253; Carbohydrates: 7g; Protein: 21g; Cholesterol: 180mg; Total Fat: 8g; Saturated Fat: 3g; Sodium: 343mg; Potassium: 554mg; Calcium: 120mg

# Shrimp Salad in Avocado Halves

Flare Soother | Fatigue-Friendly | Kidney Support | Bone Booster | Gluten-Free

Buy precooked bay shrimp at your grocery store fish counter, which saves time and makes this recipe super easy to put together. It's perfect for a light lunch, and it travels well. If you plan to take it with you for lunch, don't halve the avocado until just before you are ready to serve, to keep the avocado from browning.

**SERVES 4**
**PREP** 10 minutes
**COOK** None

2 cups cooked baby shrimp

¼ cup Easy Mayonnaise (page 195)

1 teaspoon Dijon mustard

½ teaspoon dried tarragon

¼ teaspoon sea salt

⅛ teaspoon black pepper

2 avocados, halved, pitted, and scooped out from the peel

2 tablespoons lemon juice

1. In a medium bowl, combine the shrimp, mayonnaise, mustard, tarragon, salt, and pepper until well mixed.

2. Place the avocado halves on a plate, cut-side up. Sprinkle with the lemon juice.

3. Spoon the salad into the avocado halves and serve.

Kidney Support Tip  Serve the shrimp salad in a lettuce leaf instead of an avocado half. Chop ½ avocado and scatter it on top of the shrimp salad to lower the potassium level.

PER SERVING (½ cup shrimp salad, ½ avocado) Calories: 366; Carbohydrates: 14g; Protein: 22g; Cholesterol: 183mg; Total Fat: 26g; Saturated Fat: 5g; Sodium: 451mg; Potassium: 647mg; Calcium: 108mg

# Spicy Shrimp with Sautéed Citrus Kale

Flare Soother | Fatigue-Friendly | Bone Booster | Gluten-Free

Cooking greens is simple when you're experiencing a flare-up, because they require minimal preparation, particularly if you buy a bag of pretrimmed greens. For example, you can choose bagged kale, which already has the stems and ribs trimmed away so all you get is the good stuff.

**SERVES 4**
**PREP** 10 minutes
**COOK** 20 minutes

2 tablespoons extra-virgin olive oil

12 ounces peeled, deveined shrimp

2 garlic cloves, minced

½ teaspoon sea salt

⅛ to ¼ teaspoon cayenne pepper

4 cups trimmed kale

¼ cup orange juice

1. In a large sauté pan over medium-high heat, heat the olive oil until it shimmers.

2. Add the shrimp and cook, stirring occasionally, until opaque, about 5 minutes. Add the garlic, salt, and cayenne and cook, stirring constantly, for 30 seconds. Use a slotted spoon to transfer the shrimp to a plate, and tent with aluminum foil to keep warm.

3. In the same pan, sauté the kale in the oil that remains, stirring occasionally, until it is soft, about 7 minutes.

4. Add the orange juice. Cook, stirring occasionally, for 4 minutes more.

5. Serve the shrimp arranged on top of the kale.

Flare Soother Tip Replace the cayenne with 1 teaspoon ground ginger.

Fatigue-Friendly Tip Use pretrimmed bagged kale, or replace the kale with baby spinach. Use 1 teaspoon minced garlic from a jar.

Kidney Support and Cardio Care Tip Reduce the salt to ¼ teaspoon to minimize sodium intake.

PER SERVING (3 ounces shrimp, ½ cup greens) Calories: 142; Carbohydrates: 20g; Protein: 2g; Cholesterol: 0mg; Total Fat: 7g; Saturated Fat: 1g; Sodium: 263mg; Potassium: 441mg; Calcium: 120mg

# Shrimp and Winter Squash Packets

Flare Soother | Fatigue-Friendly | Bone Booster | Gluten-Free

Cinnamon and Dijon mustard add lots of flavor to this slightly sweet shrimp dish. Using foil packets will keep the shrimp moist and allow the squash to steam in the juices.

**SERVES 4**
**PREP** 10 minutes
**COOK** 20 minutes

4 cups peeled and cubed winter squash such as butternut squash

12 ounces medium shrimp, peeled and deveined

1 tablespoon extra-virgin olive oil

½ cup orange juice

1 tablespoon Dijon mustard

1 tablespoon honey

1 teaspoon ground cinnamon

1 teaspoon onion powder

½ teaspoon garlic powder

½ teaspoon sea salt

¼ teaspoon black pepper

1. Preheat the oven to 400°F.

2. Fold four large squares of aluminum foil into packets, leaving room to fold the opening closed. Place the packets on a rimmed baking sheet.

3. Divide the squash and shrimp evenly among the packets.

4. In a small bowl, whisk together the olive oil, orange juice, mustard, honey, cinnamon, onion powder, garlic powder, salt, and pepper. Carefully pour the mixture over the squash and shrimp.

5. Seal the foil at the opening to make closed packets and bake until the shrimp is opaque and the squash soft, 15 to 20 minutes.

6. Serve in the packets to minimize cleanup.

Fatigue-Friendly Tip Use frozen chopped butternut squash.

Kidney Support and Cardio Care Tip Reduce the salt to ¼ teaspoon to minimize sodium intake.

PER SERVING (3 ounces shrimp, 1 cup squash) Calories: 212; Carbohydrates: 25g; Protein: 20g; Cholesterol: 167mg; Total Fat: 5g; Saturated Fat: <1g; Sodium: 477mg; Potassium: 577mg; Calcium: 120mg

Garlic Chicken Thighs and Kale Slaw, p. 165

# Meat and Poultry Entrées

# Turkey Piccata

Flare Soother | Fatigue-Friendly | Kidney Support | Big 8 Allergen–Free | Gluten-Free

When you pound turkey breasts really flat, they cook up in no time. To pound the turkey breast, place each piece between two pieces of plastic wrap or parchment paper and use a mallet or something with a flat-bottom surface to pound it to a thickness of about ¼ inch.

**SERVES 4**
**PREP** 10 minutes
**COOK** 12 minutes

12 ounces boneless, skinless turkey breast, cut into four pieces and pounded to ¼-inch thickness

½ teaspoon sea salt

¼ teaspoon black pepper

1 tablespoon extra-virgin olive oil

1 tablespoon capers, drained

2 garlic cloves, minced

¼ cup lemon juice

¼ cup Chicken Broth (page 192)

2 tablespoons arrowroot powder

1. Season the turkey with the salt and pepper.

2. In a large nonstick sauté pan or skillet over medium-high heat, heat the olive oil until it shimmers.

3. Add the turkey and cook until it is cooked through, about 4 minutes per side.

4. Transfer the turkey to a plate and tent with aluminum foil to keep warm.

5. Add the capers to the pan and cook, stirring, for 2 minutes. Add the garlic and cook, stirring constantly, for 30 seconds more.

6. In a small bowl, whisk the lemon juice and broth with the arrowroot powder. Pour into the pan. Cook, stirring, until the sauce thickens, about 1 minute.

7. Spoon the sauce over the cooked turkey and serve.

Fatigue-Friendly Tip Instead of pounding the turkey breast, just slice it lengthwise with a knife into thin strips, which will take about 5 minutes per side to cook. Use 1 teaspoon minced garlic from a jar.

Kidney Support and Cardio Care Tip Omit the salt and rinse the capers to minimize sodium intake.

PER SERVING (3 ounces turkey, 2 tablespoons sauce) Calories: 127; Carbohydrates: 5g; Protein: 15g; Cholesterol: 37mg; Total Fat: 5g; Saturated Fat: <1g; Sodium: 1,170 mg; Potassium: 298mg; Calcium: 12mg

# Turkey Burgers, Protein Style

Flare Soother | Kidney Support | Gluten-Free

In this burger recipe, you'll replace the buns with big lettuce leaves. Butter lettuce works especially well for wrapping your turkey burger, as the leaves are large and slightly cupped to hold the burger and toppings. You can also serve it open-faced (on a single lettuce leaf) and eat it with a fork and knife.

**SERVES 4**
**PREP** 10 minutes
**COOK** 8 minutes

12 ounces ground turkey breast

1 tablespoon gluten-free soy sauce or tamari

¼ teaspoon fish sauce

2 garlic cloves, minced

¼ teaspoon black pepper

1 tablespoon extra-virgin olive oil

½ cup Easy Mayonnaise (page 195)

2 tablespoons Dijon mustard

8 lettuce leaves

½ avocado, peeled, pitted, and cut into 8 slices

1. In a medium bowl, mix the ground turkey with the soy sauce, fish sauce, garlic, and pepper. Form the mixture into 4 patties.

2. In a large nonstick sauté pan or skillet over medium-high heat, heat the olive oil until it shimmers. Add the turkey burgers and cook, flipping once, until browned, about 4 minutes per side.

3. In a small bowl, whisk together the mayonnaise and mustard.

4. Place 1 lettuce leaf on each of four plates. Top with a turkey burger, 2 avocado slices, and 2 tablespoons of sauce. Top with the remaining lettuce leaf and serve.

Fatigue-Friendly Tip Use 1 teaspoon minced garlic from a jar. If using a knife causes issues, mash the avocado with a fork instead of slicing it.

Kidney Support and Cardio Care Tip Reduce soy sauce to ½ tablespoon to reduce sodium.

PER SERVING (3 ounces turkey, 2 tablespoons spread, 2 lettuce leaves) Calories: 372; Carbohydrates: 11g; Protein: 24g; Cholesterol: 94mg; Total Fat: 28g; Saturated Fat: 5g; Sodium: 646 mg; Potassium: 393mg; Calcium: 48mg

# Turkey and Green Bean Packets

Flare Soother | Fatigue-Friendly | Kidney Support | Big 8 Allergen–Free | Gluten-Free

Use aluminum foil to make a handy packet to keep ingredients moist and minimize after-dinner cleanup. This recipe is pretty simple and straightforward, so it's perfect for when you're experiencing a painful flare-up or reduced energy. You can also put the packets on your grill and close the lid if you don't want to cook them in the oven.

**SERVES 4**
**PREP** 5 minutes
**COOK** 25 minutes

2 cups frozen green beans

12 ounces boneless, skinless turkey breast, cut into four pieces

½ teaspoon sea salt

⅛ teaspoon black pepper

1 tablespoon dried rosemary

1 cup unsweetened applesauce

1. Preheat the oven to 400°F.

2. Fold four large squares of aluminum foil into packets, leaving room to fold the opening closed. Place the packets on a rimmed baking sheet.

3. Divide the green beans evenly among the packets.

4. Season the turkey with the salt, pepper, and rosemary and place it on the green beans in each packet. Spoon ¼ cup of applesauce over each piece of turkey.

5. Seal the foil at the opening to make closed packets and bake until the turkey is cooked through, 20 to 25 minutes.

6. Serve in the packets to minimize cleanup.

Kidney Support and Cardio Care Tip **Reduce the salt to ¼ teaspoon to minimize sodium intake.**

PER SERVING (3 ounces turkey, ½ cup green beans) Calories: 135; Carbohydrates: 15g; Protein: 16g; Cholesterol: 37mg; Total Fat: 2g; Saturated Fat: 0g; Sodium: 299 mg; Potassium: 423mg; Calcium: 48mg

# Baked Chicken Packets

Flare Soother | Fatigue-Friendly | Gluten-Free

In this recipe, the chicken and veggies are cooked and served in their own handy vessel, so you don't even need to use plates if you don't want to—you can eat it right out of the packet. That makes both prep and cleanup a snap, and you'll have dinner on the table in 30 minutes.

**SERVES 4**
**PREP** 5 minutes
**COOK** 25 minutes

2 cups frozen mixed vegetables

1 tablespoon Dijon mustard

1 tablespoon gluten-free soy sauce or tamari

1 tablespoon dried Italian seasoning

¼ teaspoon black pepper

12 ounces boneless, skinless chicken breast, cut into four pieces

1. Preheat the oven to 400°F.

2. Fold four large squares of aluminum foil into packets, leaving room to fold the opening closed. Place the packets on a rimmed baking sheet.

3. Divide the mixed veggies evenly among the packets.

4. In a small bowl, whisk together the mustard, soy sauce, Italian seasoning, and pepper. Spread one-quarter of the mixture on each piece of chicken and place the chicken on top of the vegetables.

5. Seal the foil at the opening to make closed packets and bake until the chicken is cooked through, 20 to 25 minutes.

6. Serve in the packets to minimize cleanup.

Kidney Support and Cardio Care Tip  Reduce the soy sauce to 2 teaspoons to minimize sodium intake.

PER SERVING (3 ounces chicken, ½ cup veggies) Calories: 196; Carbohydrates: 13g; Protein: 28g; Cholesterol: 65mg; Total Fat: 3g; Saturated Fat: <1g; Sodium: 356mg; Potassium: 347mg; Calcium: 72mg

# Easy Roasted Chicken

Flare Soother | Fatigue-Friendly | Kidney Support | Big 8 Allergen–Free | Gluten-Free

Roasting a chicken takes about 90 minutes, but it's all inactive time, so this is actually an easy recipe that doesn't require much actual work. If you're feeling fancy, you can add extra flavor to the chicken by stuffing a halved onion and a few sprigs of rosemary in the cavity of the chicken before roasting it in the oven.

**SERVES 6**
**PREP** 10 minutes
**COOK** 1 hour, 30 minutes

4 cups baby carrots
¾ teaspoon sea salt
1 tablespoon dried rosemary
1 tablespoon dried thyme
¾ teaspoon black pepper
1 (5-pound) chicken, giblets and neck removed

1. Preheat the oven to 350°F.

2. Scatter the carrots in the bottom of a roasting pan and set a rack over them.

3. In a small bowl, whisk together the salt, rosemary, thyme, and pepper. Rub the seasoning evenly over the outside of the chicken.

4. Place the chicken, breast-side up, on the rack in the roasting pan.

5. Roast until the chicken reaches an internal temperature of 180°F and the juices run clear when the thickest part of the thigh is pierced, 75 to 90 minutes. Let the chicken cool a bit and rest for 20 minutes before carving.

6. Serve the chicken with the roasted carrots.

Fatigue-Friendly Tip  To save energy, purchase a chicken that already has its giblets and neck removed.

Kidney Support Tip  Reduce the salt to ¼ teaspoon to minimize sodium intake.

Cardio Care Tip  Reduce the salt to ¼ teaspoon to minimize sodium intake. Remove the skin before eating to reduce fat and cholesterol.

PER SERVING (⅙ chicken, ⅔ cup carrots) Calories: 373; Carbohydrates: 7g; Protein: 66g; Cholesterol: 175mg; Total Fat: 7g; Saturated Fat: 2g; Sodium: 436mg; Potassium: 615mg; Calcium: 72mg

# Garlic Chicken Thighs and Kale Slaw

Flare Soother | Gluten-Free

These skin-on chicken thighs are roasted with peeled and halved garlic cloves. Roasting the garlic mellows and sweetens the flavor so it's really delicious. The colorful salad on the side is loaded with anti-inflammatory pumpkin seeds and pomegranate arils (seeds). You can buy pomegranate seeds in the produce section of your grocery store.

**SERVES 4**
**PREP** 5 minutes
**COOK** 40 minutes

**FOR THE CHICKEN**

2 tablespoons extra-virgin olive oil

4 chicken thighs

½ teaspoon sea salt

⅛ teaspoon black pepper

8 garlic cloves, peeled and halved lengthwise

¼ cup tarragon leaves (optional)

**TO MAKE THE CHICKEN**

1. Preheat the oven to 375°F.

2. In a large, ovenproof sauté pan, heat the olive oil over medium-high heat until it shimmers. Season the chicken thighs with the salt and pepper. Cook the chicken, skin-side down, until browned, about 5 minutes. Flip the chicken and brown 5 minutes on the other side.

3. Add the garlic to the pan, sprinkling it on and around the chicken.

4. Transfer the chicken to the preheated oven, cooking until the juices run clear, about 30 minutes.

5. Garnish with the tarragon (if using).

�➤

**FOR THE SLAW**

4 cups chopped kale
(or bagged kale salad)

½ cup shredded red cabbage

1 apple, peeled, cored,
and grated

¼ cup pumpkin seeds

¼ cup pomegranate arils

3 tablespoons extra-virgin
olive oil

1 tablespoon
balsamic vinegar

1 tablespoon grated ginger

¼ teaspoon sea salt

⅛ teaspoon black pepper

**TO MAKE THE SLAW**

1. In a large bowl, combine the kale, cabbage, apple, pumpkin seeds, and pomegranate arils.

2. In a small bowl, whisk the olive oil, vinegar, ginger, salt, and pepper. Toss with the salad.

Kidney Support and Cardio Care Tip  Reduce the salt on the chicken to ¼ teaspoon to minimize sodium intake.

PER SERVING  Calories: 583; Carbohydrates: 27g; Protein: 48g; Cholesterol: 130mg; Total Fat: 33g; Saturated Fat: 6g; Sodium: 512mg; Potassium: 929mg; Calcium: 260mg

# Quick Chicken and Broccoli Stir-Fry

Flare Soother | Fatigue-Friendly | Kidney Support | Cardio Care | Gluten-Free

Stir-fries make easy, no-fuss meals because they come together quickly and can be on your table in about 20 minutes. Serve this stir-fry with Cauliflower Rice (page 102) for a complete meal. It's quick, easy, and delicious, and if you use frozen broccoli, then there's not much chopping required.

**SERVES 4**
**PREP** 10 minutes
**COOK** 10 minutes

2 tablespoons extra-virgin olive oil

12 ounces boneless, skinless chicken breast, cut into bite-size pieces

2 cups small broccoli florets

½ yellow onion, chopped

2 cups sliced mushrooms

¼ cup Asian Stir-Fry Sauce (page 201)

2 tablespoons arrowroot powder

1. In a large nonstick sauté pan or skillet over medium-high heat, heat the olive oil until it shimmers.

2. Add the chicken, broccoli, onion, and mushrooms. Cook, stirring frequently, until the chicken is cooked, about 7 minutes.

3. In a small bowl, whisk together the stir-fry sauce and arrowroot powder. Add to the chicken. Cook, stirring constantly, until the sauce thickens, about 2 minutes. Serve warm.

Fatigue-Friendly Tip Use frozen broccoli florets, prechopped onions, and presliced mushrooms.

PER SERVING (2 cups) Calories: 226; Carbohydrates: 7g; Protein: 28g; Cholesterol: 65mg; Total Fat: 10g; Saturated Fat: 2g; Sodium: 528mg; Potassium: 474mg; Calcium: 48mg

# Bacon-Wrapped Rosemary Chicken Drumsticks

Flare Soother | Fatigue-Friendly | Kidney Support | Big 8 Allergen–Free | Gluten-Free

Wrapping drumsticks in bacon is genius. The bacon flavors the chicken as it cooks and gets crispy in the hot oven, so it makes a delicious main course that's really easy to prepare. Serve it with steamed veggies, applesauce, or a simple salad for a complete, nutritious meal.

**SERVES 4**
**PREP** 10 minutes
**COOK** 1 hour

4 chicken drumsticks

4 thin-cut bacon slices

1 teaspoon dried rosemary

1. Preheat the oven to 375°F.

2. Wrap each drumstick in a slice of bacon and place it on a rimmed baking sheet. Sprinkle with the rosemary.

3. Bake until the juices run clear, about 1 hour. Serve immediately.

Kidney Support and Cardio Care Tip Use low-sodium turkey bacon to reduce fat, cholesterol, and sodium.

PER SERVING (1 drumstick) Calories: 232; Carbohydrates: <1g; Protein: 23g; Cholesterol: 72mg; Total Fat: 15g; Saturated Fat: 5g; Sodium: 692mg; Potassium: 255mg; Calcium: 12mg

# Mustard-Rubbed Pork Tenderloin with Warm Fruit Compote

Flare Soother | Fatigue-Friendly | Kidney Support | Big 8 Allergen–Free | Gluten-Free

Use your food processor or blender to make this flavorful herb coating for pork tenderloin, and while it rests, prepare the fruit compote for a complete meal that's perfect for fall or winter.

**SERVES 4**
**PREP** 10 minutes
**COOK** 40 minutes

2 tablespoons Dijon mustard

¼ cup fresh parsley

2 tablespoons fresh thyme

2 tablespoons fresh rosemary

2 garlic cloves, minced

¼ teaspoon sea salt

¼ teaspoon black pepper

1 (1-pound) pork tenderloin

2 tablespoons extra-virgin olive oil

2 apples, peeled, cored, and chopped

2 pears, peeled, cored, and chopped

1. Preheat the oven to 400°F. Line a rimmed baking sheet with aluminum foil.

2. In a blender or food processor, combine the mustard, parsley, thyme, rosemary, garlic, salt, and pepper. Process until it forms a paste.

3. Spread the paste in an even layer all over the pork and place on the prepared baking sheet.

4. Bake until the pork reaches an internal temperature of 140°F, 20 to 30 minutes. Allow the pork to rest, tented with foil, for 20 minutes.

5. Meanwhile, heat the olive oil in a sauté pan over medium heat until it shimmers.

6. Add the apple and pears and cook, stirring occasionally, until the fruit is soft, about 10 minutes.

7. Slice the pork and spoon the compote on top. Serve.

Fatigue-Friendly Tip Use prechopped fruit (fresh or frozen) and 1 teaspoon minced garlic from a jar.

Kidney Support and Cardio Care Tip Reduce the salt to ¼ teaspoon to minimize sodium intake. Reduce the olive oil to 1 tablespoon.

PER SERVING (4 ounces pork, ½ cup fruit) Calories: 358; Carbohydrates: 34g; Protein: 31g; Cholesterol: 83mg; Total Fat: 12g; Saturated Fat: 3g; Sodium: 276mg; Potassium: 782mg; Calcium: 96mg

# Pork Chops and Applesauce

Flare Soother | Fatigue-Friendly | Kidney Support | Big 8 Allergen–Free | Gluten-Free

Using thin-cut, bone-in pork chops keeps protein levels and cooking times low, and home-made applesauce adds lots of flavor to this delicious dish. You can cook the applesauce while the pork chops bake. Both require minimal active time and tending, and you'll have dinner on the table in about 30 minutes.

**SERVES 4**
**PREP** 10 minutes
**COOK** 20 minutes

4 thin-cut bone-in pork chops, trimmed of visible fat

½ teaspoon sea salt

¼ teaspoon black pepper

½ teaspoon dried sage

4 cups peeled, cored, chopped apples

¼ cup apple juice

1 tablespoon pure maple syrup

1 teaspoon ground ginger

1 teaspoon ground cinnamon

1. Preheat the oven to 425°F.

2. Line a rimmed baking sheet with aluminum foil to minimize cleanup.

3. Put the chops on the prepared baking sheet and sprinkle them with the salt, pepper, and sage. Bake until the pork reaches an internal temperature of 140°F, 15 to 20 minutes. Rest, tented with foil, for 10 minutes.

4. Meanwhile, in a medium pot, combine the apples, apple juice, maple syrup, ginger, and cinnamon. Bring to a simmer over medium-high heat. Cook, stirring occasionally, until the apples are saucy and soft, about 20 minutes.

5. Serve the pork chops with the warm applesauce.

Fatigue-Friendly Tip **Use prechopped apples (fresh or frozen).**

Kidney Support and Cardio Care Tip **Reduce the salt to ¼ teaspoon to minimize sodium intake.**

PER SERVING (1 chop, ½ cup applesauce) Calories: 349; Carbohydrates: 20g; Protein: 20g; Cholesterol: 73mg; Total Fat: 21g; Saturated Fat: 8g; Sodium: 295mg; Potassium: 428mg; Calcium: 48mg

# Broccoli Beef Stir-Fry

Flare Soother | Fatigue-Friendly | Kidney Support | Bone Booster | Gluten-Free

The sirloin is sliced very thin for this tasty stir-fry so it cooks quickly. You can add a bit of heat with some red pepper flakes if you aren't sensitive to nightshades. Serve it alongside Cauliflower Rice (page 102) or Cauliflower Fried Rice (page 132) for a dinner that's far tastier and healthier than take-out.

**SERVES 4**
**PREP** 10 minutes
**COOK** 10 minutes

2 tablespoons extra-virgin olive oil

1 (12-ounce) sirloin steak, trimmed of visible fat and thinly sliced

4 cups broccoli florets

1 cup chopped scallions

1 cup sliced mushrooms

2 garlic cloves, minced

1 teaspoon ground ginger

1 cup orange juice

1 tablespoon gluten-free soy sauce or tamari

⅛ teaspoon red pepper flakes

1 tablespoon arrowroot powder

1. In a large nonstick sauté pan or skillet over medium-high heat, heat the olive oil until it shimmers.

2. Add the steak, broccoli, scallions, and mushrooms and cook, stirring frequently, until the meat is cooked through, about 7 minutes.

3. Add the garlic and ginger and cook, stirring constantly, for 30 seconds.

4. In a small bowl, whisk together the orange juice, soy sauce, red pepper flakes, and arrowroot powder. Add to the beef and broccoli mixture and cook, stirring constantly, until the sauce thickens, 1 to 2 minutes. Serve immediately.

Flare Soother Tip Omit the red pepper flakes if you are sensitive to nightshades.

Fatigue-Friendly Tip Use prechopped broccoli (fresh or frozen), and sliced scallions from the grocery store salad bar. Use 1 teaspoon minced ginger from a jar.

Kidney Support and Cardio Care Tip Reduce the soy sauce to ½ tablespoon. Omit the mushrooms for kidney support.

PER SERVING (2 cups) Calories: 295; Carbohydrates: 16g; Protein: 30g; Cholesterol: 76mg; Total Fat: 13g; Saturated Fat: 3g; Sodium: 318mg; Potassium: 906mg; Calcium: 72mg

# Sirloin Steak with Chimichurri

Flare Soother | Fatigue-Friendly | Kidney Support | Big 8 Allergen–Free | Gluten-Free

Chimichurri is a thick sauce similar to pesto. It's made of chopped garlic and herbs and is especially delicious on steak. This steak is super easy to make—just cook it in the oven, rest it, then slice it on the bias for a delicious main course you can serve with steamed veggies, mashed sweet potatoes, or a salad for a hearty meal.

**SERVES 4**
**PREP** 10 minutes
**COOK** 50 minutes

1 (1-pound) sirloin steak

½ teaspoon sea salt, divided

¼ teaspoon black pepper

1 cup fresh parsley

¼ cup fresh cilantro

3 garlic cloves, lightly smashed

½ cup red wine vinegar

2 tablespoons extra-virgin olive oil

½ teaspoon red pepper flakes

1. Preheat the oven to 400°F.

2. Line a rimmed baking sheet with aluminum foil for easy cleanup.

3. Place the steak on the baking sheet and season with ¼ teaspoon of salt and the pepper. Bake until the steak reaches an internal temperature of 140°F for medium-rare, about 50 minutes. Allow the steak to rest for 5 minutes, then slice it on the bias.

4. While the steak is in the oven, in a food processor or blender, combine the parsley, cilantro, garlic, vinegar, olive oil, red pepper flakes, and remaining ¼ teaspoon of salt. Process until the herbs and garlic are finely chopped.

5. Spoon the chimichurri over the sliced steak and serve.

Flare Soother Tip  Omit the red pepper flakes if you are sensitive to nightshades.

Cardio Care Tip  Reduce the olive oil to 1 tablespoon. Trim the steak of any visible fat.

PER SERVING (4 ounces steak, ¼ cup sauce) Calories: 287; Carbohydrates: 2g; Protein: 35g; Cholesterol: 101mg; Total Fat: 14g; Saturated Fat: 4g; Sodium: 320mg; Potassium: 582mg; Calcium: 36mg

# Meatloaf with Sweet and Sour Glaze

Kidney Support | Bone Booster | Gluten-Free

Meatloaf is a classic comfort food that's popular with the whole family. This version is made with extra-lean ground beef to keep fat and cholesterol low, and almond meal replaces the traditional bread crumbs to help you get the right texture. Serve alongside Sweet Potato Purée (page 105) or Cauliflower Purée (page 101) for a classic American dinner.

**SERVES 4**
**PREP** 10 minutes
**COOK** 75 minutes

2 tablespoons extra-virgin olive oil

1 yellow onion, chopped

2 garlic cloves, minced

1 pound extra-lean ground beef

1 tablespoon Dijon mustard

1 tablespoon gluten-free soy sauce or tamari

1 large egg, beaten

½ cup almond meal

1 teaspoon dried thyme

½ teaspoon sea salt

¼ teaspoon black pepper

¼ cup tomato paste

¼ cup apple cider vinegar

¼ cup pure maple syrup

1 tablespoon prepared horseradish

1. Preheat the oven to 350°F.

2. In a large nonstick sauté pan or skillet over medium-high heat, heat the olive oil until it shimmers. Cook the onion until soft, about 4 minutes. Add the garlic and cook, stirring constantly, for 30 seconds. Set aside to cool a bit.

3. In a large bowl, combine the cooled onion and garlic, ground beef, mustard, soy sauce, egg, almond meal, thyme, salt, and pepper and mix well. Press the mixture into an 8-by-4-inch loaf pan.

4. In a bowl, whisk together the tomato paste, vinegar, maple syrup, and horseradish. Spread over the top of the meatloaf.

5. Bake until the meatloaf reaches an internal temperature of 160°F, about 75 minutes. Cut into 4 slices and serve.

**Flare Soother Tip** Omit the glaze if you are sensitive to nightshades.

**Fatigue-Friendly Tip** Use 1 cup prechopped onion and 1 teaspoon minced garlic from a jar.

**Kidney Support and Cardio Care Tip** Reduce the salt to ¼ teaspoon. Replace the ground beef with ground turkey breast.

PER SERVING (4 ounces) Calories: 428; Carbohydrates: 24g; Protein: 35g; Cholesterol: 127mg; Total Fat: 22g; Saturated Fat: 5g; Sodium: 441mg; Potassium: 777mg; Calcium: 76mg

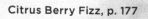
Citrus Berry Fizz, p. 177

# 10

# Drinks, Smoothies, and Desserts

# Fruit-Infused Water

Flare Soother | Fatigue-Friendly | Kidney Support | Cardio Care
Big 8 Allergen–Free | Gluten-Free

Infusing water with fruit adds flavor and nutrients, turning plain water into something really delicious. The flavor combinations you can try here are virtually endless, since you can use almost any fruits and herbs to flavor your water. For example, try combining cucumber, mint, and citrus for an invigorating beverage, or melon and basil for a lighter flavor.

**SERVES 2**
**PREP** 5 minutes,
(plus 2 hours inactive)
**COOK** None

1 cup blackberries or raspberries

2 fresh ginger slices

2 cups water

1. In a large container, combine the berries, ginger, and water.

2. Steep in the refrigerator for 2 hours before serving.

Fatigue-Friendly Tip There's no need to chop or smash the berries. The water will pull flavor from them as it rests.

PER SERVING (1 cup) Calories: 30; Carbohydrates: 7g; Protein: 1g; Cholesterol: 0mg; Total Fat: 0g; Saturated Fat: 0g; Sodium: 8mg; Potassium: 119mg; Calcium: 36mg

# Citrus Berry Fizz

Flare Soother | Kidney Support | Cardio Care | Big-8 Allergen–Free | Gluten-Free

With vitamin C from the citrus and antioxidants from the berries, this healthy and delicious drink makes a great mocktail or just a refreshing beverage any time you feel like having something a little different. Feel free to change up the citrus or berries you use to vary the flavors.

**SERVES 1**
**PREP** 5 minutes
**COOK** None

4 blackberries

4 blueberries

2 tablespoons lime juice

8 ounces sparkling water

Ice

1 basil sprig (optional)

1. In a large glass, muddle the berries with the lime juice.

2. Add the sparkling water and ice. Garnish with the basil (if using).

Flare Soother Tip  Add ¼ teaspoon of ground ginger to fight inflammation.

PER SERVING Calories: 23; Carbohydrates: 4g; Protein: <1g; Cholesterol: 0mg; Total Fat: 0g; Saturated Fat: 0g; Sodium: 11mg; Potassium: 85mg; Calcium: 48mg

# Ginger-Lemon Tea

Flare Soother | Fatigue-Friendly | Kidney Support | Cardio Care
Big 8 Allergen–Free | Gluten-Free

Ginger is a powerful anti-inflammatory ingredient, so this delicious tea is ideal when you're experiencing pain from a flare-up of inflammation. You can add other herbs or spices as desired to change the flavor profile.

**SERVES 1**
**PREP** 5 minutes
**COOK** 5 minutes

2 fresh ginger slices
1 cup boiling water
1 tablespoon honey
2 tablespoons lemon juice

1. In a large mug, steep the ginger in the water for 5 minutes (or longer, for a stronger ginger flavor).

2. Stir in the honey and lemon juice and serve hot.

Flare Soother Tip **Replace the lemon juice with orange juice, which is also a delicious anti-inflammatory ingredient.**

PER SERVING (1 cup) Calories: 71; Carbohydrates: 18g; Protein: <1g; Cholesterol: 0mg; Total Fat: 0g; Saturated Fat: 0g; Sodium: 14mg; Potassium: 51mg; Calcium: 12mg

# Quick Hot Chocolate

Flare Soother | Fatigue-Friendly | Kidney Support | Cardio Care
Big 8 Allergen–Free | Gluten-Free

If you've got a chocolate craving, this easy hot chocolate is the perfect solution.
Use unsweetened chocolate and add honey or pure maple syrup to suit your own
level of sweetness, then add other flavorings like mint or cinnamon to suit your
taste preferences.

**SERVES 1**
**PREP** 5 minutes
**COOK** 5 minutes

¼ cup unsweetened
cocoa powder

1 cup unsweetened nut milk
such as almond milk or lite
coconut milk

2 tablespoons pure
maple syrup

¼ teaspoon pure
vanilla extract

In a small saucepan, whisk together the cocoa powder, milk,
syrup, and vanilla over medium heat until warm and combined.
Serve hot.

Bone Booster Tip Replace the nut milk with skim milk to boost
calcium, but remember using dairy means it is no longer
allergen-free.

PER SERVING (1 cup) Calories: 284; Carbohydrates: 47g; Protein: 7g;
Cholesterol: 0mg; Total Fat: 14g; Saturated Fat: 12g; Sodium: 65mg;
Potassium: 411mg; Calcium: 60mg

# Chia Vanilla Milk Shake

Flare Soother | Fatigue-Friendly | Kidney Support | Big 8 Allergen–Free | Gluten-Free

With the omega-3 fatty acids in the chia, this milk shake is a delicious flare soother. Choose any type of dairy or nondairy milk that works for you. If you need calcium, for instance, choose skim milk. If you need to lower fat intake, choose almond milk. If you are allergic to nuts, choose lite coconut milk.

**SERVES 1**
**PREP** 5 minutes
**COOK** None

1 cup unsweetened nut milk such as almond milk or lite coconut milk

2 tablespoons honey

1 teaspoon pure vanilla extract

2 tablespoons chia seeds

¼ teaspoon ground nutmeg

1 cup crushed ice

In a blender, combine all the ingredients. Blend until smooth. Serve immediately.

Cardio Care Tip  Use almond milk instead of lite coconut milk to reduce saturated fat.

Bone Booster Tip  Replace the nut milk with skim milk to boost calcium, but remember using dairy means it is no longer allergen-free.

PER SERVING (1⅛ cups) Calories: 344; Carbohydrates: 47g; Protein: 6g; Cholesterol: 0mg; Total Fat: 16g; Saturated Fat: 11g; Sodium: 63mg; Potassium: 144mg; Calcium: 12mg

# Orange Creamsicle Smoothie

Flare Soother | Fatigue-Friendly | Kidney Support | Big 8 Allergen–Free | Gluten-Free

The flaxseed meal in this smoothie increases anti-inflammatory omega-3 fatty acids, which makes it a great inflammation soother when combined with the vitamin C from the oranges and the nutritious minerals in the coconut milk.

**SERVES 2**
**PREP** 5 minutes
**COOK** None

1½ cups orange juice

1 cup lite coconut milk

1 teaspoon pure
vanilla extract

2 tablespoons flaxseed meal

1 cup crushed ice

In a blender, combine all the ingredients. Blend until smooth. Serve immediately.

Cardio Care Tip **Use almond milk instead of lite coconut milk to reduce saturated fat.**

Bone Booster Tip **Replace the lite coconut milk with skim milk to boost calcium, but remember using dairy means it is no longer allergen-free.**

PER SERVING (1⅛ cups) Calories: 195; Carbohydrates: 26g; Protein: 4g; Cholesterol: 0mg; Total Fat: 9g; Saturated Fat: 6g; Sodium: 34mg; Potassium: 432mg; Calcium: 0mg

# Pumpkin Pie Smoothie

Flare Soother | Fatigue–Friendly | Kidney Support | Big 8 Allergen–Free | Gluten–Free

Pumpkin is an excellent source of anti-inflammatory vitamin A, and it has a delicious, earthy flavor that makes this smoothie taste a lot like pumpkin pie. Flaxseed meal, ginger, cinnamon, and nutmeg further fight inflammation, making this a great smoothie to have when you're experiencing a flare-up. Be sure to use pumpkin purée, not pumpkin pie filling.

**SERVES 2**
**PREP** 5 minutes
**COOK** None

1½ cups pumpkin purée

2 tablespoons flaxseed meal

½ teaspoon ground ginger

½ teaspoon ground cinnamon

¼ teaspoon ground nutmeg

2 cups unsweetened nut milk such as lite coconut milk or almond milk

1 cup crushed ice

In a blender, combine all the ingredients. Blend until smooth. Serve immediately.

**Cardio Care Tip** Use almond milk instead of lite coconut milk to reduce saturated fat.

**Bone Booster Tip** Replace the nut milk with skim milk to boost calcium, but remember using dairy means it is no longer allergen-free.

PER SERVING (1⅛ cups) Calories: 239; Carbohydrates: 27g; Protein: 6g; Cholesterol: 0mg; Total Fat: 15g; Saturated Fat: 12g; Sodium: 71mg; Potassium: 445mg; Calcium: 72mg

# Almond, Flax, and Chocolate Smoothie

Flare Soother | Fatigue-Friendly | Kidney Support | Gluten-Free

Almond butter is an excellent source of healthy fats and vitamin E, while flaxseed meal supplies anti-inflammatory omega-3 fatty acids. With the protein from the almond butter, this smoothie makes a great meal replacement when you're not feeling up to (or don't have time for) working in the kitchen. This recipe is high in potassium, so if you have kidney issues it's best to avoid it.

**SERVES 1**
**PREP** 5 minutes
**COOK** None

1½ cups lite coconut milk

2 tablespoons honey

1 tablespoon almond butter

¼ cup unsweetened cocoa powder

2 tablespoons flaxseed meal

1 cup crushed ice

In a blender, combine all the ingredients. Blend until smooth. Serve immediately.

Cardio Care Tip **Use almond milk instead of lite coconut milk to reduce saturated fat.**

Bone Booster Tip **Replace the lite coconut milk with skim milk to boost calcium.**

PER SERVING (1⅛ cups) Calories: 529; Carbohydrates: 90g; Protein: 11g; Cholesterol: 0mg; Total Fat: 20g; Saturated Fat: 3g; Sodium: 140mg; Potassium: 686mg; Calcium: 72mg

# Coconut Pudding

Flare Soother | Fatigue-Friendly | Cardio Care | Bone Booster
Big 8 Allergen–Free | Gluten-Free

This creamy pudding makes a delicious, refreshing dessert. It needs to chill for a few hours in the refrigerator before you serve it, so be sure to plan ahead when you make it. Canned lite coconut milk has enough coconut flavor to bring it to the forefront in this silky-smooth pudding.

**SERVES 4**
**PREP** 5 minutes
**COOK** 5 minutes

2 cups lite coconut milk, divided

¼ cup honey

Pinch sea salt

3 tablespoons arrowroot powder

1. In a small saucepan, heat 1½ cups of coconut milk, the honey, and salt over medium-high heat, stirring constantly. Bring it to a boil.

2. In a small bowl, whisk together the remaining ½ cup of coconut milk and the arrowroot powder. Stir this mixture slowly into the hot coconut milk mixture. Boil for 1 minute, stirring constantly.

3. Refrigerate for 2 hours before serving.

Flare Soother Tip **Add 1 teaspoon ground ginger to boost anti-inflammatory properties.**

PER SERVING (½ cup) Calories: 136; Carbohydrates: 23g; Protein: 2g; Cholesterol: 0mg; Total Fat: 6g; Saturated Fat: 6g; Sodium: 71mg; Potassium: 37mg; Calcium: 0mg

# Date Bonbons

Flare Soother | Fatigue-Friendly | Kidney Support | Cardio Care
Big 8 Allergen–Free | Gluten-Free

These come together quickly in a blender or food processor, and they make a tasty sweet treat for when you're craving chocolate. Made without any refined sugar and with nutrient-dense ingredients, this is a healthy dessert you'll be happy to serve to your family.

**SERVES 6**
**PREP** 10 minutes
**COOK** None

2 tablespoons honey

¼ cup unsweetened cocoa powder

1 cup pitted Medjool dates

½ cup unsweetened coconut flakes

1. In a blender or food processor, combine all the ingredients. Process until smooth.

2. Roll the mixture into 6 balls. Refrigerate for at least 1 hour to firm up before serving.

Flare Soother Tip  Add ½ teaspoon ground ginger or 1 teaspoon grated fresh ginger to boost anti-inflammatory properties.

PER SERVING (1 bonbon) Calories: 137; Carbohydrates: 31g; Protein: 2g; Cholesterol: 0mg; Total Fat: 3g; Saturated Fat: 2g; Sodium: 3mg; Potassium: 277mg; Calcium: 24mg

# Easy Almond Butter Cookies

Flare Soother | Fatigue-Friendly | Cardio Care | Gluten-Free

These cookies don't contain any processed ingredients like sugar or flour, but they're still delicious and fragrant as you bake them. They are sure to become a family favorite, and they're high in vitamin E and protein, so they make a great sweet treat. Freeze them in a zip-top bag for up to six months.

**SERVES 12**
**PREP** 10 minutes
**COOK** 12 minutes

1 cup chunky almond butter

⅓ cup pure maple syrup

1 large egg, beaten

1 teaspoon pure vanilla extract

½ teaspoon baking soda

Pinch sea salt

1. Preheat the oven to 350°F.

2. Line a baking sheet with parchment paper or aluminum foil.

3. In a bowl, beat together all the ingredients until smooth.

4. Drop the dough in 1-tablespoon mounds on the prepared baking sheet. Bake until done, 10 to 12 minutes. Cool on a wire rack.

Kidney Support Tip  Almonds are fairly high in potassium, so the key here is portion control. One cookie won't hurt. A dozen will provide too much potassium.

PER SERVING (1 cookie) Calories: 37; Carbohydrates: 6g; Protein: <1g; Cholesterol: 14mg; Total Fat: 1g; Saturated Fat: 0g; Sodium: 78mg; Potassium: 33mg; Calcium: 12mg

# Chocolate-Covered Frozen Bananas

Flare Soother | Fatigue-Friendly | Big 8 Allergen–Free | Gluten-Free

Looking for a tasty, simple treat? Look no further than bananas dipped in a sweet chocolate shell and then frozen. It's a quick, easy, and delicious dessert. The bananas will take about six hours to freeze, so make them ahead of time to have them ready for dessert. You'll need four ice pop sticks to make these.

**SERVES 4**
**PREP** 10 minutes
**COOK** None

4 ounces unsweetened chocolate

1 tablespoon coconut oil

2 packets stevia

2 bananas, peeled and halved

1. Line a large plate with parchment paper or aluminum foil.

2. In a small saucepan, melt the chocolate, coconut oil, and stevia over low heat, stirring constantly.

3. Insert a stick in the cut end of each banana half. Dip the bananas in the chocolate and set on the prepared plate. Freeze for 6 hours before serving.

Kidney Support Tip Half a banana is high in potassium, but as long as you watch your potassium intake the rest of the day, this sweet treat won't cause much harm.

PER SERVING (½ banana) Calories: 224; Carbohydrates: 21g; Protein: 4g; Cholesterol: 0mg; Total Fat: 18g; Saturated Fat: 12g; Sodium: 7mg; Potassium: 447mg; Calcium: 36mg

# Easy Chocolate Mousse

Flare Soother | Fatigue-Friendly | Big 8 Allergen–Free | Gluten-Free

This ridiculously easy dessert takes less than 10 minutes to make and doesn't require any cooking. It's perfect for an after-dinner treat when you're craving chocolate.

**SERVES 4**
**PREP** 10 minutes
**COOK** None

2 avocados, peeled and pitted

¼ cup unsweetened cocoa powder

½ cup lite coconut milk

1 teaspoon pure vanilla extract

¼ cup pure maple syrup

1. In a blender or food processor, combine all the ingredients. Process until smooth.

2. Serve immediately or refrigerate for later.

Kidney Support Tip **Use portion control if you have kidney issues, because avocados are high in potassium.**

Ingredient Tip **Add the zest of 1 orange to add a delicious citrus flavor.**

PER SERVING (½ cup) Calories: 289; Carbohydrates: 26g; Protein: 3g; Cholesterol: 0mg; Total Fat: 22g; Saturated Fat: 6g; Sodium: 17mg; Potassium: 611mg; Calcium: 36mg

# Apple Blueberry Crumble

Flare Soother | Gluten-Free

This easy apple and blueberry crumble has a sweet nut topping and a delicious fruit filling. You make the filling on the stove top, and then broil the crumble lightly for a nutritious fruit dessert that's easy to make and really tasty.

**SERVES 4**
**PREP** 15 minutes
**COOK** 15 minutes

**FOR THE FRUIT FILLING**

2 tablespoons coconut oil

4 sweet-tart apples such as Honeycrisp, peeled, cored, and chopped

3 tablespoons pure maple syrup

½ teaspoon cinnamon

½ teaspoon ground ginger

¼ teaspoon nutmeg

Pinch sea salt

1 cup blueberries

**FOR THE CRUMBLE**

½ cup finely chopped pecans

½ cup finely chopped hazelnuts

3 tablespoons ground flaxseed

¼ cup pure maple syrup

½ teaspoon cinnamon

⅛ teaspoon sea salt

**TO MAKE THE FRUIT FILLING**

1. In a large saucepan over medium-high heat, heat the coconut oil.

2. Add the apples and cook, stirring occasionally, for 5 minutes.

3. Add the syrup, cinnamon, ginger, nutmeg, salt, and blueberries. Cook, stirring frequently, for 5 minutes more.

4. Spoon the mixture into four 8-ounce ramekins.

**TO MAKE THE CRUMBLE**

1. Set the broiler to high heat.

2. In a small bowl, combine all ingredients.

3. Spoon the mixture over the fruit mixture in the ramekins.

4. Broil for 2 to 3 minutes to brown the topping.

Cardio and Kidney Support Tip To minimize sodium, eliminate the salt altogether.

PER RAMEKIN Calories: 472; Carbohydrates: 65g; Protein: 7g; Cholesterol: 0mg; Total Fat: 24g; Saturated Fat: 7g; Sodium: 124mg; Potassium: 532mg; Calcium: 60mg

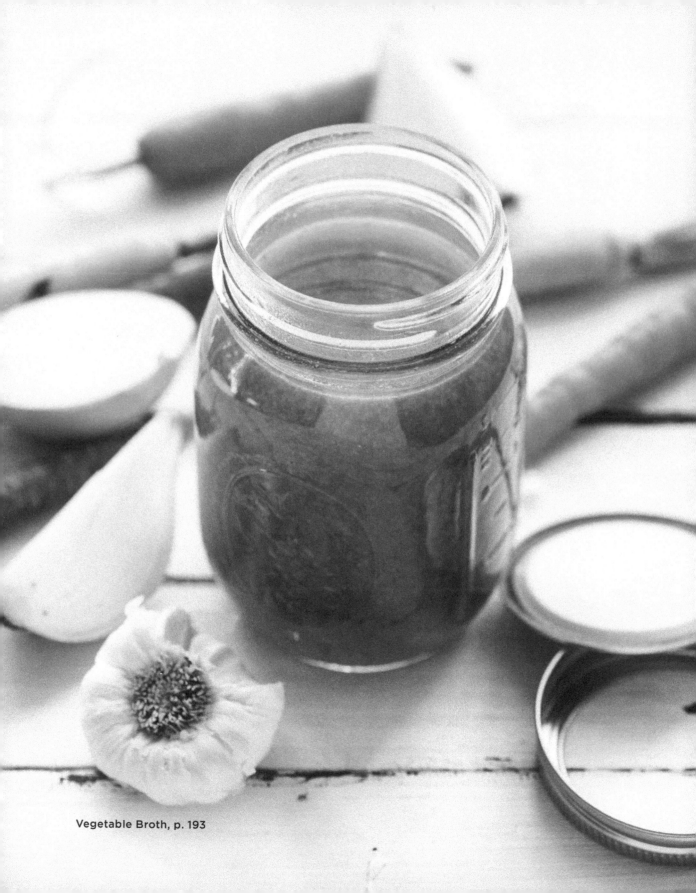

Vegetable Broth, p. 193

# 11

# Broths, Sauces, and Dressings

# Chicken Broth

Flare Soother | Fatigue-Friendly | Kidney Support | Cardio Care
Bone Booster | Big 8 Allergen–Free | Gluten-Free

This chicken broth serves as the base for many of the recipes in this cookbook. While the method calls for making it on the stove top, you can also put all the ingredients in a slow cooker and cook on low for 12 to 24 hours. The longer you cook the broth, the more minerals seep into it. Don't cook for more than 24 hours in a slow cooker, though, or it may get bitter. Freeze the broth in 1-cup servings for up to a year so you'll always have it on hand for recipes.

**MAKES 6 CUPS**
**PREP** 5 minutes
**COOK** 3 hours

2 pounds meaty chicken bones such as necks, backs, and wings

2 carrots, cut into four pieces each

1 yellow onion, cut into four pieces

2 celery stalks, cut into four pieces each

1 teaspoon dried rosemary

1 teaspoon dried thyme

8 peppercorns

10 cups water

1. In a large pot, combine all the ingredients. Simmer over medium-low heat for 3 hours (or longer).

2. Strain the solids from the broth and discard them.

Flare Soother Tip Chicken feet add a lot of gelatin to broth, which is excellent for soothing inflammation. If you can find chicken feet, add one or two to the broth as it cooks.

Ingredient Tip Feel free to use turkey parts instead of chicken.

PER SERVING (1 cup) Calories: 15; Carbohydrates: 1g; Protein: 2g; Cholesterol: 0mg; Total Fat: 0g; Saturated Fat: 0g; Sodium: 35mg; Potassium: 0mg; Calcium: 0mg

# Vegetable Broth

Fatigue-Friendly | Kidney Support | Cardio Care | Bone Booster
Big 8 Allergen–Free | Gluten-Free

You can cook this in a large pot on the stove top or in a slow cooker for up to 24 hours. The broth is made without salt to minimize sodium. Store the broth in 1-cup servings in the freezer for up to a year to use as needed. Thaw in the refrigerator, on the stove top, or in the microwave for a minute or two.

**MAKES 6 CUPS**
**PREP** 5 minutes
**COOK** 3 hours

4 carrots, quartered

4 celery stalks, quartered

2 yellow onions, quartered

8 ounces mushrooms

1 teaspoon dried rosemary

1 teaspoon dried thyme

8 peppercorns

6 garlic cloves

10 cups water

1. In a large pot, combine all the ingredients. Simmer over medium-low heat for 3 hours (or longer).

2. Strain the solids from the broth and discard them.

Fatigue-Friendly Tip There's no need to spend much time chopping the veggies. You can cut them in half just so they fit in the pot, and the water will still extract the flavors. Since you'll be straining away the solids, you don't even need to peel the onions and carrots as long as you cut them in half.

PER SERVING (1 cup) Calories: 15; Carbohydrates: 1g; Protein: 2g; Cholesterol: 0mg; Total Fat: 0g; Saturated Fat: 0g; Sodium: 35mg; Potassium: 0mg; Calcium: 0mg

# Mushroom Broth

Fatigue-Friendly | Kidney Support | Cardio Care | Bone Booster
Big 8 Allergen–Free | Gluten-Free

Using dried mushrooms adds intense savory flavor to broth, which in turn adds tremen-dous flavor to the dishes you cook using it. You can use any type of dried mushrooms here, although if you can find them, porcini mushrooms add the richest flavor. You can find dried mushrooms in the produce section at the grocery store.

**MAKES 2 CUPS**
**PREP** 5 minutes
**COOK** 5 minutes
(plus 3 hours inactive)

2 cups Vegetable Broth
(page 193) or Chicken Broth
(page 192)

2 ounces dried mushrooms

1. In a saucepan, combine the broth and mushrooms and bring to a boil over high heat.

2. Turn off the heat, cover the pot, and allow the mushrooms to steep in the broth for 3 hours.

3. Strain the mushrooms from the broth and discard them.

Fatigue-Friendly Tip Save time by making mushroom broth when you make your other broth. Strain 2 cups of the hot broth and pour it over the mushrooms. There's no need to bring it to a boil—the hot broth will extract the flavor from the mushrooms.

PER SERVING (1 cup) Calories: 15; Carbohydrates: 1g; Protein: 2g; Cholesterol: 0mg; Total Fat: 0g; Saturated Fat: 0g; Sodium: 35mg; Potassium: 0mg; Calcium: 0mg

# Easy Mayonnaise

Fatigue-Friendly | Kidney Support | Cardio Care | Bone Booster | Gluten-Free

Making mayonnaise is easy if you have a blender or food processor, and homemade mayo is much more nutritious than the stuff you buy in a jar, which may contain high fructose corn syrup, sugar, or artificial ingredients. This version is made with minimal salt, so it doesn't add sodium to your recipes.

**MAKES ABOUT 1 CUP**
**PREP** 5 minutes
**COOK** None

1 large egg yolk

1 teaspoon Dijon mustard

1 tablespoon lemon juice

1 tablespoon red
wine vinegar

Pinch salt

1 cup extra-virgin olive oil

1. In a blender or food processor, combine the egg yolk, mustard, lemon juice, vinegar, and salt.

2. With the blender or food processor running on high, add a drip of oil, followed by another drip. Then, add the remaining oil in a thin stream.

Ingredient Tip Some people find the flavor of extra-virgin olive oil too strong in this mayonnaise. If that's the case for you, use half olive oil and half avocado oil.

PER SERVING (1 tablespoon) Calories: 112; Carbohydrates: <1g; Protein: <1g; Cholesterol: 13mg; Total Fat: 13g; Saturated Fat: 2g; Sodium: 14mg; Potassium: 4mg; Calcium: 0mg

# Easy Tartar Sauce

Fatigue-Friendly | Kidney Support | Gluten-Free

Tartar sauce in a jar can be pretty high in sodium. This fresh version tastes better than the commercial stuff—and it's healthier for you. You can serve this tartar sauce with many of the seafood recipes in this book.

**MAKES ABOUT 1 CUP**
**PREP** 10 minutes
**COOK** None

1 cup Easy Mayonnaise
(page 195)

1 dill pickle, finely chopped

1 scallion, finely chopped

1 tablespoon chopped
fresh parsley

1 tablespoon lemon juice

1 teaspoon Dijon mustard

Pinch salt

Pinch red pepper flakes

In a small bowl, whisk together all the ingredients.

**Flare Soother Tip** If you are sensitive to nightshades, omit the red pepper flakes.

**Fatigue-Friendly Tip** Instead of chopping the pickles, parsley, and onion by hand, pulse them a few times in a food processor or blender.

**Cardio Care Tip** To reduce fat and cholesterol, replace half of the mayonnaise with ½ cup fat-free plain yogurt.

PER SERVING (2 tablespoons) Calories: 117; Carbohydrates: 8g; Protein: <1g; Cholesterol: 8mg; Total Fat: 10g; Saturated Fat: 2g; Sodium: 335mg; Potassium: 16mg; Calcium: 12mg

# Lemon-Basil Vinaigrette

Flare Soother | Fatigue-Friendly | Kidney Support | Big 8 Allergen–Free | Gluten-Free

A well-made vinaigrette consists of three parts oil and one part acid, plus a pinch salt, a teaspoon of mustard to help emulsify it, and your choice of herbs and spices. With that formula in mind, you can take this basic vinaigrette recipe and make your own variations based on your favorite flavors.

**MAKES ABOUT 1 CUP**
**PREP** 5 minutes
**COOK** None

¾ cup extra-virgin olive oil

2 tablespoons lemon juice

2 tablespoons apple cider vinegar

1 teaspoon Dijon mustard

1 teaspoon garlic powder

1 teaspoon dried basil

Pinch salt

In a small bowl, whisk together all the ingredients until emulsified.

**Flare Soother Tip** Replace the dried basil with ½ teaspoon ground ginger or 1 teaspoon grated fresh ginger, and replace the lemon juice with orange juice.

**Fatigue-Friendly Tip** If you're not up for whisking, combine all the ingredients in a jar and shake to combine.

**Cardio Care Tip** For a lower-fat dressing, double the lemon juice and apple cider vinegar to ¼ cup each, and use only ¼ cup olive oil.

PER SERVING (2 tablespoons) Calories: 165; Carbohydrates: <1g; Protein: <1g; Cholesterol: 0mg; Total Fat: 19g; Saturated Fat: 3g; Sodium: 28mg; Potassium: 13mg; Calcium: 0mg

# Honey Mustard Dressing

Fatigue-Friendly | Kidney Support | Gluten-Free

Using homemade Easy Mayonnaise (page 195) as a base, it's a breeze to whip up this dressing in no time at all. Along with being a delicious dressing for Cobb Salad (page 88), it's also tasty on meat, fish, or poultry or as a dip for raw veggies. It will keep in the refrigerator for up to a week.

**MAKES ABOUT ½ CUP**
**PREP** 5 minutes
**COOK** None

6 tablespoons Easy Mayonnaise (page 195)

2 tablespoons Dijon mustard

2 tablespoons honey

In a small bowl, whisk together all the ingredients until combined.

**Cardio Care and Bone Booster Tip** If you're not sensitive to dairy, replace the mayonnaise with fat-free plain yogurt to add calcium and minimize fat.

PER SERVING (2 tablespoons) Calories: 123; Carbohydrates: 14g; Protein: <1g; Cholesterol: 6mg; Total Fat: 8g; Saturated Fat: 1g; Sodium: 120mg; Potassium: 18mg; Calcium: 12mg

# Creamy Avocado Dressing

Flare Soother | Fatigue-Friendly | Kidney Support | Cardio Care
Big 8 Allergen–Free | Gluten-Free

You can whip up this tasty dressing in the blender in a matter of minutes. With anti-inflammatory ingredients and healthy fats, it's a great topper for coleslaw, salad, or even seafood, poultry, or meat. You can also try this as a dip for Baked Sweet Potato Wedges (page 98). Avocados are a bit high in potassium, but as long as you limit your serving sizes, it won't be an issue for kidney support.

**MAKES ABOUT 1 CUP**
**PREP** 5 minutes
**COOK** None

1 avocado, peeled and pitted
¼ cup fresh cilantro
¼ cup apple cider vinegar
¼ cup lime juice
1 teaspoon ground ginger
1 teaspoon garlic powder
⅛ teaspoon sea salt
⅛ teaspoon black pepper

In a small blender or food processor, process all the ingredients until smooth.

Bone Booster Tip Replace the avocado with ½ cup fat-free plain yogurt to boost calcium if you are not sensitive to dairy, but remember using dairy means it is no longer allergen-free.

PER SERVING (2 tablespoons) Calories: 57; Carbohydrates: 3g; Protein: <1g; Cholesterol: 0mg; Total Fat: 5g; Saturated Fat: 1g; Sodium: 35mg; Potassium: 147mg; Calcium: 12mg

# Ginger-Garlic Vinaigrette

Flare Soother | Fatigue-Friendly | Kidney Support | Cardio Care
Big 8 Allergen–Free | Gluten-Free

This vinaigrette variation makes a tasty marinade or delicious salad dressing. The ginger is anti-inflammatory, and honey adds a touch of sweetness without being overpowering. If salt isn't an issue for you, you can adjust the seasoning levels to your own personal preferences.

**MAKES ABOUT 1 CUP**
**PREP** 5 minutes
**COOK** None

¾ cup extra-virgin olive oil

¼ cup apple cider vinegar

2 garlic cloves, minced

1 tablespoon honey

1 teaspoon Dijon mustard

1 teaspoon grated
fresh ginger

¼ teaspoon sea salt

¼ teaspoon black pepper

In a small bowl, whisk together all the ingredients until combined.

Fatigue-Friendly Tip Use 1 teaspoon minced garlic from a jar or tube. You might also be able to find tubes of minced ginger in the produce section of your grocery store. Don't use garlic powder or ground ginger, because they lack the flavor necessary to make this vinaigrette bright.

PER SERVING (2 tablespoons) Calories: 174; Carbohydrates: 3g; Protein: <1g; Cholesterol: 0mg; Total Fat: 19g; Saturated Fat: 3g; Sodium: 66mg; Potassium: 13mg; Calcium: 0mg

# Asian Stir-Fry Sauce

Flare Soother | Fatigue-Friendly | Gluten-Free

Whether you're using meat, poultry, seafood, or veggies, try this sauce the next time you make a stir-fry. It has lots of anti-inflammatory ginger, and orange juice adds vitamin C. This also makes a good marinade for meats, poultry, and seafood, so it's easy and versatile.

**MAKES ABOUT ½ CUP**
**PREP** 5 minutes
**COOK** None

½ cup orange juice

2 tablespoons gluten-free soy sauce or tamari

2 tablespoons honey

1 teaspoon ground ginger

1 teaspoon garlic powder

Pinch red pepper flakes (optional)

In a small bowl, whisk together all the ingredients until combined.

Flare Soother Tip  Eliminate the red pepper flakes if you are sensitive to nightshades.

Kidney Support and Cardio Care Tip  To minimize sodium, use only 1 tablespoon low-sodium soy sauce.

PER SERVING (2 tablespoons) Calories: 54; Carbohydrates: 13g; Protein: <1g; Cholesterol: 0mg; Total Fat: <1g; Saturated Fat: 0g; Sodium: 452mg; Potassium: 100mg; Calcium: 0mg

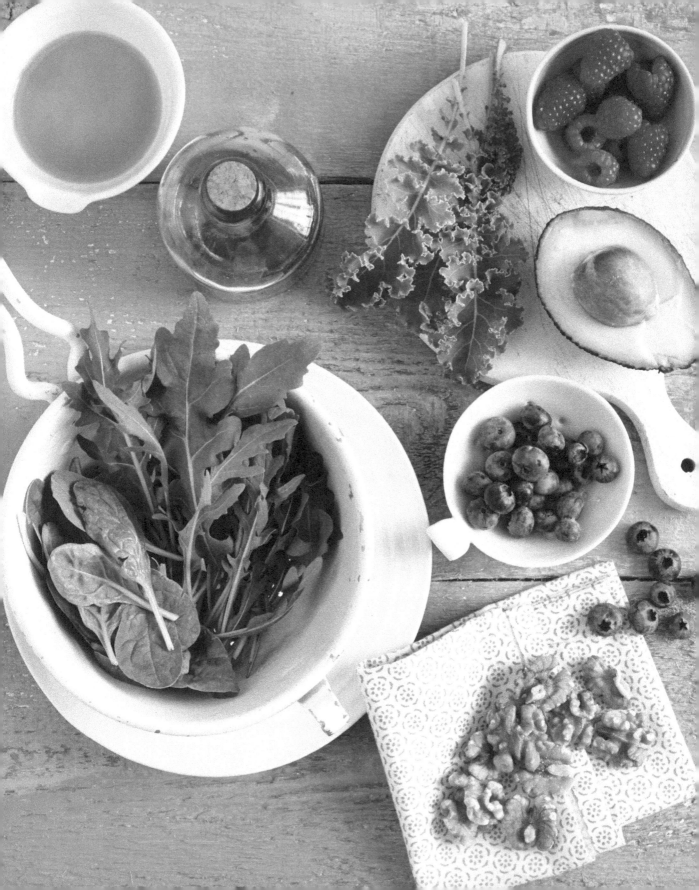

# Acknowledgments

I would like to express my appreciation to the countless individuals who have helped with this book—thanks to everyone who provided support, wrote, read, offered comments, and assisted in editing, proofreading, and design.

I am especially grateful to the Callisto Media team for enabling me to pursue my passion and vocation to further educate and inform those affected by lupus. Special thanks go to Karen Frazier for her assistance in the development of the recipes.

*"Life is too short. If there was ever a moment to follow your passion and do something that matters to you, that moment is now."*

—Unknown author

# Resources

**The American Autoimmune Related Diseases Association** (aarda.org) brings a national focus to autoimmunity, the major cause of many serious chronic diseases, including lupus. The website provides the latest news and research, financial tools, and information on autoimmune disease.

**The Lupus Foundation of America** website (lupus.org) contains a wealth of useful information about current research, support groups with lists of local chapters, and frequently asked questions associated with lupus.

**The Lupus Research Alliance** (lupusresearchinstitute.org) is a nonprofit devoted to research on lupus. Breakthroughs in research have been made in determining the genetics of lupus, why and how certain organs get attacked in lupus, details about the autoimmune response, and biomarkers of lupus development.

**Molly's Fund Fighting Lupus** (mollysfund.org) was started in 2005 in order to help educate, advocate, inform, and support the public about lupus. The website contains information on local and online support groups as well as information on financial assistance programs.

**The National Institute of Arthritis and Musculoskeletal and Skin Diseases** website (niams.nih.gov) offers the latest publications, research, events, and more on causes, treatment, and prevention of arthritis and musculoskeletal and skin diseases, including those associated with lupus.

*The First Year—Lupus* is a book written by patient expert Nancy Hanger, which walks you through everything you need to learn about lupus during the first year after your diagnosis.

Amazon Prime Pantry (amazon.com)

Herbs Pro (herbspro.com)

Retail Me Not (retailmenot.com)

Thrive Market (thrivemarket.com)

Vitacost (vitacost.com)

# References

## Books

Aladjem, Henrietta. *The Challenges of Lupus: Insights and Hope.* Garden City Park, NY: Avery Publishing Group, 1998.

Hanger, Nancy C., and Andrea B. Schneebaum. *The First Year—Lupus: An Essential Guide for the Newly Diagnosed.* New York: Da Capo Press, 2003.

Lahita, Robert G., and Robert H. Phillips. *Lupus: Everything You Need to Know.* Garden City Park, NY: Avery Publishing Group, 1998.

Wallace, David J. *The Lupus Book: A Guide for Patients and Their Families.* 5th ed. New York: Oxford University Press, 2012.

## Articles

Bogaczewicz, Jaroslaw, Elzbieta Karczmarewicz, Pawel Pludowski, Jakub Zabek, Jan Kowalski, Jacek Lukaszkiewicz, and Anna Wozniacka. "Feasibility of Measurement of Bone Turnover Markers in Female Patients with Systemic Lupus Erythematosus." *Revista Brasileira de Reumatologia* 55, no. 2 (March–April 2015): 133–39. doi:10.1016/j.rbr.2014.10.004.

Borges, Mariane Curado, Fabiana de Miranda Moura Santos, Rosa Weiss Telles, Maria Isabel Toulson Davisson Correia, and Cristina Costa Duarte Lanna. "Polyunsaturated Omega-3 Fatty Acids and Systemic Lupus Erythematosus: What Do We Know?" *Revista Brasileira de Reumatologia* 54, no. 6 (November–December 2014): 459–66. doi:10.1016/j.rbr.2013.12.002.

Boyle, Aimee. "Stretching: The Mental Health Benefits." EmpowHer. Accessed December 28, 2016. www.empowher.com/lupus/content/stretching-mental-health-benefits.

Brown, Amy C. "Lupus Erythematosus and Nutrition: A Review of the Literature." *Journal of Renal Nutrition* 10, no. 4 (October 2000): 170–83.

Cohen, Sheldon, Denise Janicki-Deverts, William J. Doyle, Gregory E. Miller, Ellen Frank, Bruce S. Rabin, and Ronald B. Turner. "Chronic Stress, Glucocorticoid Receptor Resistance, Inflammation, and Disease Risk." *Proceedings of the National Academy of Science of the United States of America* 109, no. 16 (February 2012): 5995–99.

DiChiara, Tom. "Can Exercise at Night Hurt Your Sleep?" CNN. April 22, 2014. www.cnn.com/2014/04/22/health/upwave-night-exercise/.

Everett, Sotiria. "Nutrition and Lupus Part 1: Ways to Maintain a Healthy Diet." Hospital for Special Surgery. January 28, 2010. www.hss.edu/conditions_nutrition-and-lupus-part1.asp.

Gut Microbiota News Watch. "A Study Establishes New Connections between Gut Microbiota and Autoimmune Diseases." January 20, 2015. www.gutmicrobiota forhealth.com/en/a-study-establishes -new-connections-between-gut-microbiota -and-autoimmune-diseases/.

Hanson, Rick. "Confronting the Negativity Bias." *Rick Hanson, Ph.D.* October 26, 2010. www.rickhanson.net /how-your-brain-makes-you -easily-intimidated/.

Hardy, Carolyn J., Benedict P. Palmer, Kenneth R. Muir, Alex J. Sutton, and Richard J. Powell. "Smoking History, Alcohol Consumption, and Systemic Lupus Erythematosus: A Case-Control Study." *Annals of the Rheumatic Diseases* 57, no. 8 (1998): 451–55.

Healthline. "List of Common Lupus Medications." Accessed November 25, 2016. www.healthline.com/health/lupus /medications-list#Othermedications4.

Iliades, Chris. "The Benefits in Exercise in Lupus Management." Everyday Health. April 6, 2009. www.everydayhealth.com/lupus /lupus-benefits-of-exercise.aspx.

Iliades, Chris. "Managing Your Diet to Keep Lupus In Control." Everyday Health. April 6, 2009. www.everydayhealth.com/lupus /manage-diet-to-control-lupus.aspx.

Khansari, Nemat, Yadollah Shakiba, and Mahdi Mahmoudi. "Chronic Inflammation and Oxidative Stress as a Major Cause of Age-Related Diseases and Cancer." *Recent Patents on Inflammation and Drug Discovery* 3, no. 1 (January 2009): 73–80.

Klack, Karin, Eloisa Bonfa, and Eduardo Ferreira Borba Neto. "Diet and Nutritional Aspects in Systemic Lupus Erythematosus." *Revista Brasileira de Reumatologia* 52, no. 3 (May–June 2012): 395–408. doi:10.1590 /S0482-50042012000300009.

Leech, Barbara. "Helpful, Energizing Foods for Lupus." New Life Outlook. May 7, 2014. lupus.newlifeoutlook.com/fueling-energy/.

Ludlam, Kerry. "Exercises for Lupus." WebMD.com. Accessed December 11, 2016. www.webmd.com/lupus/features /lupus-exercise#1.

Lupus Foundation of America. "15 Questions: Healthy Eating." June 2011. www.lupus.org /resources/15-questions-healthy-eating.

Lupus Foundation of America. "How Is Remission in Lupus Defined?" July 18, 2013. www.lupus.org/answers/entry /how-is-remission-in-lupus-defined.

Lupus Foundation of America. "Statistics on Lupus." June 2016. www.lupus.org/about /statistics-on-lupus.

Lupus Foundation of America. "What Medications are Used to Treat Lupus?" July 12, 2013. www.lupus.org/answers/entry /medications-to-treat-lupus.

Lupus Foundation of Minnesota. "Types of Lupus." Accessed November 24, 2016. www .lupusmn.org/what-is-lupus/types-of-lupus/.

Lupus Research Alliance. "Diagnosis Lupus: Next Steps." Accessed November 24, 2016. www.lupusny.org/about-lupus/newsletters /diagnosis-lupus-next-steps.

Lupus Research Alliance. "Saturated Fats May Increase Inflammation, According to New Study." September 8, 2015. www.lupus researchinstitute.org/lupus-news/2015 /09/08/saturated-fats-may-increase -inflammation-according-new-study.

Lupus Research Alliance. "Steroids and Weight Gain." Accessed November 25, 2016. www.lupusny.org/about-lupus/newsletters /march-april-2006/steroids-and-weight-gain.

Marshall, Tess. "21 Tips to Release Self-Neglect and Love Yourself in Action." Tiny Buddha. Accessed December 19, 2016. tinybuddha.com /blog/21-tips-to-release-self-neglect-and-love -yourself-in-action/.

Mayo Clinic. "Lupus: Complications." November 18, 2014. www.mayoclinic.org /diseases-conditions/lupus/basics /complications/CON-20019676.

Mayo Clinic. "Prednisone and Other Cortico-steroids." November 26, 2015. www.mayo clinic.org/steroids/art-20045692.

Medina-Quiñones, Carmen V., Lucía Ramos-Merino, Pablo Ruiz-Sada, and David Isenberg. "Analysis of Complete Remission in Systemic Lupus Erythematosus Patients Over a 32-Year Period." *Arthritis Care and Research* 68, no. 7 (July 2016): 981–87. doi:10.1002 /acr.22774.

Minami, Yuko, Takeshi Sasaki, Yumiko Arai, Yoko Kurisu, and Shigeru Hisamichi. "Diet and Systemic Lupus Erythematosus: A 4-Year Prospective Study of Japanese Patients." *Journal of Rheumatology* 30, no 4. (April 2003): 747–54.

Mu, Qinghui, Husen Zhang, and Xin M. Luo. "SLE: Another Autoimmune Disorder Influ-enced by Microbes and Diet?" *Frontiers in Immunology* 6, no. 608 (November 2013).

National Institute of Arthritis and Musculo-skeletal and Skin Diseases. "Handout on Health: Systemic Lupus Erythematosus." June 2016. www.niams.nih.gov/health_info /lupus/.

National Institute of Arthritis and Musculo-skeletal and Skin Diseases. "Understanding Autoinflammatory Diseases." March 2016. www.niams.nih.gov/health_info /autoinflammatory/.

National Institute of Arthritis and Musculo-skeletal and Skin Diseases. "Vitamin A and Anti-Inflammatory Activity." June 2008. www.niams.nih.gov/News_and_Events /Spotlight_on_Research/2008/VitaminA _Anti_Inflam.asp.

National Sleep Foundation. "Healthy Sleep Tips." Accessed December 10, 2016. sleepfoundation.org/sleep-tools-tips /healthy-sleep-tips.

Noble, Breana. "Lupus and Probiotics: Is There a Hidden Link?" *Newsmax.* January 6, 2016. www.newsmax.com/FastFeatures /lupus-probiotics/2016/01/06/id/708470/.

Office on Women's Health. "Lupus Fact Sheet." July 16, 2012. www.womenshealth .gov/publications/our-publications /fact-sheet/lupus.html.

Palter, Jenny Thorn. "Sleep Easy: Why Sleep Is Critical When You Have Lupus." Lupus Foundation of America. July 1, 2010. www .lupus.org/magazine/entry/sleep-easy.

Ruperto, N., L. M. Hanrahan, G. S. Alarcón, H. M. Belmont, R. L. Brey, P. Brunetta, J. P. Buyon, M. I. Costner, M. E. Cronin, M. A. Dooley, et al. "International Consensus for a Definition of Disease Flare in Lupus." *Lupus* 20, no. 5 (April 2011): 453–62.

Stothers, Sarah. "Five Things People with Lupus Should Know Before Starting a Spring-time Exercise Routine." Lupus Foundation of America. March 11, 2014. www.lupus.org /blog/entry/5-things-people-with-lupus -should-know-before-starting-an-exercise -routine.

University of Texas at Austin. "Self-Esteem." Accessed December 19, 2016. cmhc.utexas .edu/selfesteem.html.

Urowitz, Murray B., Marie Feletar, Ian N. Bruce, Dominique Ibanez, and Dafna D. Gladman. "Prolonged Remission in Systemic Lupus Erythematosus." *Journal of Rheumatology* 32, no. 8 (August 2005): 1467–72.

Wallace, Daniel J. "Patient Education: Systemic Lupus Erythematosus." UpToDate. January 10, 2017. www.uptodate.com /contents/systemic-lupus-erythematosusa -sle-beyond-the-basics.

Wilson, Timothy. "Can't Help Myself: Review of *The Power of Habit,* by Charles Duhigg." New York Times. March 9, 2012. www .nytimes.com/2012/03/11/books/review /the-power-of-habit-by-charles-duhigg.html.

Wu, Tianfu, Chun Xie, Jie Han, Yujin Ye, Jim Weiel, Quan Li, Irene Blanco, et al. "Metabolic Disturbances Associated with Systemic Lupus Erythematosus." *Public Library of Science* 7, no 7 (June 2012): doi:10.1371/journal .pone.0037210.

Zhang, Husen, Xiaofeng Liao, Joshua B. Sparks, and Xin M. Luo. "Dynamics of Gut Microbiota in Autoimmune Lupus." *Applied and Environmental Microbiology* 80, no. 24 (December 2014): 7551–60.

# Meal Plan Pantry and Shopping Lists

The following lists may help you prepare for the meal plans in this book. You don't always need to purchase every item on the list. For example, some people like to stick with one or two oils when they cook, and others may find that one or two vinegars are sufficient for all of the recipes. Swap ingredients to fit your budget and taste.

Before you go shopping, review the recipes in the meal plan with these lists and decide whether or not you want to prepare all of the recipes in the meal plan. If you don't think a recipe looks appealing, then you can skip it (and cross its ingredients off the shopping list) and make extras of another recipe instead. This will also keep costs down and prevent you from wasting money on ingredients that you may not use very often.

## Basic Lupus Meal Plan Shopping List

### PANTRY

- Allspice, ground
- Almond butter
- Almond flour
- Arrowroot powder
- Baking soda
- Basil, dried
- Chia seeds
- Chili powder
- Chocolate, unsweetened
- Cinnamon, ground
- Cloves, ground
- Cocoa powder, unsweetened
- Coconut flakes, unsweetened
- Coconut flour
- Coconut oil
- Cooking spray
- Coriander, ground
- Cumin, ground
- Curry powder
- Fish sauce
- Flaxseed meal
- Garlic powder
- Ginger, ground
- Honey
- Horseradish, prepared
- Italian seasoning
- Maple syrup, pure
- Mustard, Dijon
- Nutmeg, ground
- Oil, olive, extra-virgin
- Oil, sesame, toasted
- Oil, walnut
- Onion powder
- Oregano, dried
- Paprika, smoked
- Paprika, sweet
- Pepper, black, ground
- Pepper, cayenne
- Peppercorns, black
- Red pepper flakes
- Rosemary, dried

- Sage, dried
- Salsa
- Sea salt
- Sesame seeds
- Sriracha
- Stevia
- Tahini
- Tamari, gluten-free
- Tarragon, dried
- Thyme, dried
- Turmeric, ground
- Vanilla extract, pure
- Vinegar, apple cider
- Vinegar, balsamic
- Vinegar, red wine
- Vinegar, rice
- Vinegar, white

## WEEK 1

### PRODUCE

- Apple juice (8 ounces)
- Apples (8)
- Apples, dried (1 cup)
- Apricots, dried (¼ cup)
- Asparagus (8 ounces)
- Avocados (2)
- Bananas (8)
- Blueberries (3 pints)
- Broccoli (2 large bunches)
- Carrots (14)
- Cauliflower (1 head)
- Celery (2 bunches)
- Garlic (1 bulb)
- Ginger, fresh (1 large knob)
- Grapes (1 cup)

- Kale (1 bunch)
- Lemons (3)
- Lettuce, romaine (3 heads)
- Mushrooms, button (1 pound)
- Mushrooms, dried (2 ounces)
- Mushrooms, portobello (8)
- Onions, yellow (6)
- Orange juice (10 ounces)
- Peas, fresh or frozen (1 pound)
- Potatoes, red (2)
- Salad mix (8 ounces)
- Scallions (9)
- Spinach, baby (8 ounces)
- Squash, yellow (1 medium)
- Strawberries (1 pint)
- Sweet potato (1)
- Swiss chard (1 bunch)
- Tomatoes (4 large)
- Zucchini (3 medium)

### DAIRY AND EGGS

- Cheddar, low-fat (4 ounces)
- Eggs (2 dozen)
- Milk, almond (1 quart)
- Milk, skim (1 gallon)
- Yogurt, plain (24 ounces)

### MEAT

- Bacon, thin-sliced (8 ounces)
- Beef, sirloin (12 ounces)
- Chicken, meaty bones (backs or wings) (2 pounds)
- Pork, chops (thin-cut, bone-in) (4)
- Salmon (12 ounces)
- Turkey bacon (8 ounces)
- Turkey, ground breast (12 ounces)
- Chicken, rotisserie (1)

## FROZEN

- Blueberries (8 ounces)
- Spinach (2 cups thawed)

## CANNED

- Artichoke hearts (1 [14-ounce] can)
- Clams, chopped (2 [4-ounce] cans)
- Coconut milk, full-fat (1 [14-ounce] can)
- Coconut milk, lite (1 [14-ounce] can)
- Lentils (1 [14-ounce] can)
- Oranges, mandarin (1 [4-ounce] can)
- Pumpkin purée (1 [14 ounce] can)
- Tomatoes, diced (1 [14-ounce] can)
- Tuna, water-packed (5 [5-ounce] cans)

## NUTS AND SEEDS

- Almonds, sliced (1 cup)
- Pumpkin seeds, hulled (1 pound)
- Walnuts, shelled (1 cup)

## WEEK 2

### PRODUCE

- Apple juice (24 ounces)
- Apples (3)
- Apples, dried (¼ cup)
- Apricots, dried (¼ cup)
- Avocados (6)
- Bananas (5)
- Blueberries (1 pint)
- Broccoli (1 large bunch)
- Brussels sprouts (1 pound)
- Carrots (8)
- Carrots, baby (1 pound)
- Cauliflower (1 head)
- Celery (6 stalks)
- Cilantro (1 bunch)
- Coleslaw mix (12 ounces)

- Dates, Medjool (1 cup)
- Garlic (2 bulbs)
- Jicama (1)
- Kale (2 bunches)
- Lemons (3)
- Lettuce, romaine (1 head)
- Limes (3)
- Mangoes (2)
- Mushrooms, button (24 ounces)
- Onion, red (1)
- Onions, yellow (7)
- Oranges (4)
- Parsley (1 bunch)
- Pears (2)
- Peas, fresh or frozen (8 ounces)
- Potatoes, white (2 medium)
- Raspberries (1 pint)
- Scallions (6)
- Spinach, baby (28 ounces)
- Sweet potatoes (3)
- Swiss chard (1 bunch)
- Zucchini (2 medium)

### DAIRY AND EGGS

- Butter, unsalted (4 ounces)
- Eggs (2 dozen)
- Milk, almond (1 pint)
- Milk, skim (½ gallon)
- Yogurt, plain (16 ounces)

### MEAT

- Beef, ground, extra-lean (1 pound)
- Beef, sirloin (1 pound)
- Canadian bacon (8 slices)
- Chicken, breast (boneless, skinless) (12 ounces)
- Chicken, meaty bones (backs, wings) (4 pounds)

- Chicken, rotisserie (1)
- Chicken, whole roaster (1)
- Fish, white (cod, halibut) (12 ounces)
- Salmon (12 ounces)
- Shrimp, baby (cooked) (1½ pounds)
- Turkey bacon (8 ounces)
- Turkey, ground breast (1 pound)

### CANNED

- Chiles, chopped green (1 [2-ounce] can)
- Coconut milk, lite (2 [14-ounce] cans)
- Seltzer (8 ounces)
- Tomato paste (4 ounces)
- White beans (2 [14-ounce] cans)

### NUTS AND SEEDS

- Almonds, sliced (8 ounces)
- Pumpkin seeds, hulled (8 ounces)
- Walnuts, raw (1 pound)

## WEEK 3

### PRODUCE

- Apples (3)
- Apples, dried (¼ cup)
- Apricots, dried (¼ cup)
- Avocados (3)
- Bananas (7)
- Bell pepper, red (1)
- Blueberries (2 pints)
- Carrots (11)
- Cauliflower (1 head)
- Celery (1 bunch)
- Cilantro (1 bunch)
- Coleslaw mix (1 [1-pound] bag)
- Garlic (2 bulbs)
- Lemons (2)
- Limes (3)

- Mushrooms, button (1 pound)
- Onions, yellow (6)
- Orange juice (4 ounces)
- Parsley (1 bunch)
- Pears (2)
- Peas, fresh or frozen (2 cups)
- Raspberries (1 pint)
- Rosemary (1 bunch)
- Scallions (3)
- Spinach, baby (4 ounces)
- Strawberries (1 pint)
- Sweet potatoes (4)
- Thyme (1 bunch)
- Zucchini (7 medium)

### DAIRY AND EGGS

- Eggs (1 dozen)
- Milk, almond (½ pint)
- Milk, skim (1 gallon)
- Yogurt, plain (16 ounces)

### MEAT

- Bacon, thin-sliced (8 ounces)
- Beef, ground, extra-lean (10 ounces)
- Chicken, drumsticks (4)
- Chicken, meaty bones (backs, wings) (4 pounds)
- Cod (12 ounces)
- Fish, white (cod, halibut) (12 ounces)
- Pork, tenderloin (1 pound)
- Turkey bacon (8 ounces)
- Turkey, breast (boneless, skinless) (12 ounces)

### FROZEN

- Blueberries (1 cup)
- Mixed vegetables (2 cups)

### CANNED

- Applesauce, unsweetened (4 ounces)
- Black beans (1 [14-ounce] can)
- Capers (2 ounces)
- Coconut milk (lite) (3 [14-ounce] cans)
- Pumpkin purée (1 [14-ounce] can)
- Tomatoes and green chiles, diced (such as Ro-Tel) (1 [14-ounce] can)

### NUTS AND SEEDS

- Almonds (4 ounces)
- Almonds, sliced (1 cup)
- Pumpkin seeds, hulled (8 ounces)
- Walnuts (1 cup)

## WEEK 4

### PRODUCE

- Apples (3)
- Apples, dried (2 ounces)
- Apricots, dried (2 ounces)
- Avocados (3)
- Bananas (5)
- Blueberries (3 pints)
- Carrots (12)
- Celery (4 stalks)
- Garlic (1 bulb)
- Jicama (1)
- Kale (3 bunches)
- Lemons (4)
- Lime (1)
- Mushrooms (1 pound)
- Onions, yellow (5)
- Orange juice (12 ounces)
- Oranges (2)
- Peaches (2)
- Plums (2)
- Raspberries (1 pint)
- Spinach, baby (8 ounces)
- Squash, butternut (1)
- Strawberries (1 pint)
- Sweet potatoes (2)
- Zucchini (5)

### DAIRY AND EGGS

- Eggs (2 dozen)
- Milk, almond (½ gallon)
- Yogurt, plain (24 ounces)

### MEAT

- Canadian bacon (8 slices)
- Chicken, meaty bones (backs, wings) (4 pounds)
- Cod (12 ounces)
- Salmon (12 ounces)
- Shrimp, medium (12 ounces)
- Turkey bacon (8 ounces)
- Turkey, breast (boneless, skinless) (12 ounces)
- Turkey jerky, low-sodium (4 ounces)
- White fish (cod, halibut) (12 ounces)

### FROZEN

- Carrots, chopped (3 cups)
- Green beans (2 cups)

### CANNED

- Applesauce, unsweetened (8 ounces)
- Black beans (2 [14-ounce] cans)
- Chiles, chopped green (1 [2-ounce] can)
- Coconut milk, lite (3 [14-ounce] can)

- Almonds (2 ounces)
- Almonds, sliced (1 cup)
- Pumpkin seeds, hulled (8 ounces)
- Walnuts (1 cup)

# Flare Soother Meal Plan

### PANTRY

- Allspice, ground
- Almond butter
- Almond flour
- Arrowroot powder
- Baking soda
- Basil, dried
- Chia seeds
- Chocolate, unsweetened
- Cinnamon, ground
- Cloves, ground
- Cocoa powder, unsweetened
- Coconut flakes, unsweetened
- Coconut flour
- Coconut milk (canned)
- Coconut oil
- Cooking spray
- Coriander, ground
- Cumin, ground
- Curry powder
- Fish sauce
- Flaxseed meal
- Garlic, minced (in a jar in the produce section)
- Garlic powder
- Ginger, ground
- Ginger, fresh (in a tube in the produce section)
- Honey

- Horseradish, prepared
- Italian seasoning
- Lemon juice
- Lime juice
- Maple syrup, pure
- Mustard, Dijon
- Nutmeg, ground
- Oil, olive, extra-virgin
- Oil, sesame, toasted
- Oil, walnut
- Onion powder
- Oregano, dried
- Pepper, black, ground
- Peppercorns, black
- Rosemary, dried
- Sage, dried
- Sea salt
- Sesame seeds
- Stevia
- Tahini
- Tamari, gluten-free
- Tarragon, dried
- Thyme, dried
- Turmeric, ground
- Vanilla extract, pure
- Vinegar, apple cider
- Vinegar, balsamic
- Vinegar, red wine
- Vinegar, rice
- Vinegar, white

## WEEK 1

### PRODUCE

- Apple juice (8 ounces)
- Apples (6)
- Apples, dried (½ cup)
- Apricots, dried (½ cup)

- Avocados (2)
- Bananas (7)
- Blueberries (4 pints)
- Broccoli (2 bunches)
- Carrots (12)
- Cauliflower (1 head)
- Celery (1 bunch)
- Garlic, minced (1 jar)
- Garlic (1 bulb)
- Ginger, chopped (in a tube)
- Grapes (1 cup)
- Kale (1 bunch)
- Lettuce, romaine (3 heads)
- Mushrooms, button (24 ounces)
- Mushrooms, dried (2 ounces)
- Mushrooms, portobello (8)
- Onions, yellow (8)
- Orange juice (8 ounces)
- Raspberries (1 pint)
- Salad mix (2 [8-ounce] bags)
- Scallions (12)
- Spinach, baby (10 ounces)
- Squash, yellow (1)
- Strawberries (1 pint)
- Sweet potato (1)
- Swiss chard (1 bunch)
- Zucchini (6 medium)

### DAIRY AND EGGS

- Cheese, cheddar, grated (4 ounces)
- Eggs (2 dozen)
- Milk, almond (½ gallon)
- Yogurt, plain (24 ounces)

### MEAT

- Beef, sirloin (12 ounces)
- Chicken, rotisserie (1)
- Clam meat, fresh or canned (4 ounces)
- Chicken, meaty bones (backs, wings) (2 pounds)
- Pork, thin-cut chops (4)
- Turkey bacon (8 ounces)
- Turkey, ground breast (12 ounces)

### FROZEN

- Blueberries (8 ounces)
- Peas (8 ounces)
- Spinach (1 pound)

### CANNED

- Artichoke hearts (1 [14-ounce] can)
- Asparagus (8 ounces)
- Beets, pickled (1 [14-ounce] can)
- Coconut milk, full-fat (1 [14-ounce] can)
- Coconut milk, lite (4 [14-ounce] cans)
- Lentils (1 [14-ounce] can)
- Oranges, mandarin (1 [4-ounce] can)
- Pumpkin purée (1 [14-ounce] can)
- Tuna, low-sodium, water-packed (4 [5-ounce] cans)

### NUTS AND SEEDS

- Pumpkin seeds, hulled (4 ounces)
- Walnuts (2 ounces)

## WEEK 2

### PRODUCE

- Apple juice, unsweetened (16 ounces)
- Apples (4)
- Apples, dried (½ cup)
- Apricots, dried (½ cup)
- Avocados (5)
- Bananas (3)
- Blueberries (2 pints)
- Brussels sprouts (1 pound)

- Carrots (7)
- Cauliflower (1 head)
- Celery (5)
- Cilantro (1 bunch)
- Coleslaw mix (10 ounces)
- Dates, Medjool (1 cup)
- Garlic (1 bulb)
- Kale (1 bunch)
- Lemon (1)
- Mushrooms, button (8 ounces)
- Mushrooms, sliced (2 cups)
- Onion, red (1)
- Onions, yellow (9)
- Orange juice (16 ounces)
- Parsley (1 bunch)
- Pears (3)
- Raspberries (2 pints)
- Salad greens (20 ounces)
- Spinach, baby (10 ounces)
- Sweet potatoes (6)
- Zucchini (4)

### DAIRY AND EGGS

- Eggs (2 dozen)
- Milk, almond (1 quart)
- Yogurt, plain (16 ounces)

### MEAT

- Beef, ground (1 pound)
- Beef, sirloin (1 pound)
- Canadian bacon (8 slices)
- Chicken, breast (boneless, skinless)
- Chicken, rotisserie (1)
- Salmon (12 ounces)
- Shrimp, baby (cooked) (1 pound)
- Turkey bacon (8 ounces)
- Turkey, ground breast (1 pound)
- White fish (cod, halibut) (12 ounces)

### FROZEN

- Broccoli (12 ounces)
- Mangoes (12 ounces)
- Peas (8 ounces)

### CANNED

- Coconut milk, lite (8 [14-ounce] cans)
- Sparkling water (8 ounces)
- White beans (2 [14-ounce] cans)

### NUTS AND SEEDS

- Pumpkin seeds, hulled (6 ounces)

## WEEK 3

### PRODUCE

- Apple juice, unsweetened (8 ounces)
- Apples (4)
- Apples, dried (½ cup)
- Apricots, dried (½ cup)
- Avocados (4)
- Bananas (8)
- Blueberries (3 pints)
- Carrots (16)
- Carrots, baby (2 pounds)
- Cauliflower (1 head)
- Celery (8)
- Cilantro (1 bunch)
- Coleslaw mix (1 [1-pound] bag)
- Dates, Medjool (1 cup)
- Garlic (2 bulbs)
- Kale (1 bunch)
- Mushrooms, button (24 ounces)
- Onions, yellow (7)
- Orange juice (8 ounces)
- Parsley (1 bunch)
- Pears (3)

- Raspberries (2 pints)
- Rosemary (1 bunch)
- Scallions (3)
- Spinach, baby (10 ounces)
- Strawberries (1 pint)
- Sweet potatoes (4)
- Swiss chard (1 bunch)
- Thyme (1 bunch)
- Zucchini (9)

### DAIRY AND EGGS

- Eggs (2 dozen)
- Milk, almond (½ gallon)
- Yogurt, plain (32 ounces)

### MEAT

- Bacon, thin-sliced (8 ounces)
- Beef, ground, extra-lean (10 ounces)
- Chicken, drumsticks (4)
- Chicken, meaty bones (backs, wings) (4 pounds)
- Chicken, whole roaster (1)
- Cod (12 ounces)
- Fish, white (cod, halibut) (12 ounces)
- Pork, tenderloin (1 pound)
- Salmon (12 ounces)
- Turkey bacon (8 ounces)
- Turkey, breast (boneless, skinless) (12 ounces)

### FROZEN

- Blueberries (4 ounces)
- Mixed vegetables (1 pound)
- Peas (8 ounces)

### CANNED

- Applesauce, unsweetened (8 ounces)
- Black beans (1 [14-ounce] can)
- Capers (1 ounce)
- Chickpeas (1 [14-ounce] can)
- Coconut milk (4 [14-ounce] cans)
- Pumpkin purée (1 [14-ounce] can)

### NUTS AND SEEDS

- Pumpkin seeds, hulled (4 ounces)
- Walnuts (4 ounces)

## WEEK 4

### PRODUCE

- Apple juice, unsweetened (8 ounces)
- Apples (6)
- Apples, dried (½ cup)
- Apricots, dried (½ cup)
- Avocados (3)
- Bananas (3)
- Blueberries (2 pints)
- Carrots (4)
- Celery (2)
- Garlic (1 bulb)
- Lemon (1)
- Lime (1)
- Kale (3 bunches)
- Mushrooms (8 ounces)
- Onions, yellow (4)
- Orange juice (12 ounces)
- Peaches (2)
- Plums (2)
- Raspberries (1 pint)
- Spinach, baby (10 ounces)
- Squash, butternut (1)
- Strawberries (1 pint)
- Zucchini (6)

### DAIRY AND EGGS

- Eggs (2 dozen)
- Milk, almond (½ gallon)
- Yogurt, plain (16 ounces)

### MEAT

- Canadian bacon (8 ounces)
- Fish, white (cod, halibut) (12 ounces)
- Pork, thin-cut chops (4)
- Shrimp, medium (12 ounces)
- Trout (1 pound)
- Turkey bacon (8 ounces)
- Turkey jerky, low-sodium (2 ounces)

### FROZEN

- Blueberries (8 ounces)
- Carrots, chopped (1 pound)
- Green beans (1 pound)

### CANNED

- Black beans (2 [14-ounce] cans)
- Coconut milk, lite (3 [14-ounce] cans)
- Pumpkin purée (1 [14-ounce] can)

### NUTS AND SEEDS

- Almonds, slivered (2 ounces)
- Pumpkin seeds, hulled (6 ounces)
- Walnuts (4 ounces)

## Kidney Support Meal Plan

### PANTRY

- Allspice, ground
- Almond butter
- Almond flour
- Arrowroot powder

- Baking soda
- Basil, dried
- Chia seeds
- Chili powder
- Chocolate, unsweetened
- Cinnamon, ground
- Cloves, ground
- Cocoa powder, unsweetened
- Coconut flakes, unsweetened
- Coconut flour
- Coconut milk (canned)
- Coconut oil
- Cooking spray
- Coriander, ground
- Cumin, ground
- Curry powder
- Fish sauce
- Flaxseed meal
- Garlic powder
- Ginger, ground
- Honey
- Horseradish, prepared
- Italian seasoning
- Maple syrup, pure
- Mustard, Dijon
- Nutmeg, ground
- Oil, olive, extra-virgin
- Oil, sesame, toasted
- Oil, walnut
- Onion powder
- Oregano, dried
- Paprika, smoked
- Paprika, sweet
- Pepper, black, ground
- Pepper, cayenne
- Peppercorns, black
- Red pepper flakes
- Rosemary, dried

- Sage, dried
- Salsa
- Sea salt
- Sesame seeds
- Sriracha
- Stevia
- Tahini
- Tamari, gluten-free
- Tarragon, dried
- Thyme, dried
- Turmeric, ground
- Vanilla extract, pure
- Vinegar, apple cider
- Vinegar, balsamic
- Vinegar, red wine
- Vinegar, rice
- Vinegar, white

## WEEK 1

### PRODUCE

- Apples (10)
- Apples, dried (½ cup)
- Asparagus (18 ounces)
- Avocado (½)
- Banana (1)
- Blueberries (3 pints)
- Broccoli (2 large bunches)
- Carrots (11)
- Cauliflower (1 head)
- Celery (6)
- Garlic (2 bulbs)
- Ginger, fresh (1 knob)
- Grapes (1 cup)
- Jicama
- Kale (2 bunches)
- Lemons (2)

- Lettuce, romaine (1 head)
- Mushrooms, button (1 pound)
- Mushrooms, dried (2 ounces)
- Mushrooms, portobello (8)
- Onions, yellow (8)
- Orange juice (12 ounces)
- Pear (1)
- Raspberries (2 pints)
- Salad greens (2 [10-ounce] bags)
- Scallions (14)
- Spinach, baby (1 [10-ounce] bag)
- Squash, yellow (1 medium)
- Sweet potatoes (2)
- Swiss chard (1 bunch)
- Zucchini (4 medium)

### DAIRY AND EGGS

- Cheese, low-fat (4 ounces)
- Eggs (2 dozen)
- Milk, almond (½ gallon)
- Yogurt, plain (32 ounces)

### MEAT

- Bacon, low-sodium, reduced-fat (8 ounces)
- Beef, sirloin (12 ounces)
- Chicken, meaty bones (backs, wings) (4 pounds)
- Chicken, rotisserie (1)
- Pork, thin-cut chops (4)
- Salmon (12 ounces)
- Tuna, low-sodium, water-packed (3 [5-ounce] cans)
- Turkey, breast, ground (12 ounces)

### FROZEN

- Peas (24 ounces)
- Spinach (12 ounces)

### CANNED

- Artichoke hearts (1 [14-ounce] can)
- Clams (1 [4-ounce] can)
- Coconut milk, full-fat (1 [14-ounce] can)
- Coconut milk, lite (2 [14-ounce] cans)
- Oranges, mandarin (4 ounces)
- Pumpkin purée (1 [14-ounce] can)
- Tomatoes, diced, low-sodium
  (1 [14-ounce] can)

### NUTS AND SEEDS

- Pumpkin seeds, hulled (4 ounces)

## WEEK 2

### PRODUCE

- Apples (4)
- Apples, dried (½ cup)
- Avocado (1)
- Bell pepper, green (1)
- Bell pepper, orange (1)
- Bell pepper, red (1)
- Bell pepper, yellow (1)
- Blackberries (1 pint)
- Blueberries (2 pints)
- Broccoli (3 large bunches)
- Celery (4)
- Carrots (6)
- Carrots, baby (1 pound)
- Cauliflower (2 heads)
- Cilantro (1 bunch)
- Coleslaw mix (1 [10-ounce] bag)
- Dates, Medjool (1 cup)
- Garlic (1 bulb)
- Ginger, fresh (1 large knob)
- Lemons (2)
- Limes (3)

- Mangoes (2)
- Mushrooms, button (12 ounces)
- Onion, red (1)
- Onions, yellow (8)
- Orange juice (16 ounces)
- Pears (2)
- Raspberries (3 pints)
- Salad greens (2 [10-ounce] bags)
- Scallions (13)
- Spinach, baby (1 pound)
- Squash, spaghetti (1)
- Strawberries (1 pint)
- Sweet potatoes (3)
- Zucchini (5 medium)

### DAIRY AND EGGS

- Eggs (3 dozen)
- Milk, almond (½ gallon)
- Yogurt, plain (16 ounces)

### MEAT

- Bacon, low-sodium, reduced-fat (4 ounces)
- Beef, sirloin (12 ounces)
- Chicken, breast (boneless, skinless)
  (12 ounces)
- Chicken, meaty bones (backs, wings)
  (4 pounds)
- Chicken, rotisserie (1)
- Fish, white (cod, halibut) (12 ounces)
- Shrimp, baby (cooked) (1 pound)
- Turkey, ground breast (2 pounds)

### CANNED

- Coconut milk, lite (7 [14-ounce] cans)
- Kidney beans (1 [14-ounce] can)
- Seltzer (8 ounces)
- Tomato paste (4 ounces)

### NUTS AND SEEDS

- Pumpkin seeds, hulled (4 ounces)

## WEEK 3

### PRODUCE

- Apples (3)
- Apples, dried (½ cup)
- Avocado (1)
- Blueberries (2 pints)
- Carrots (8)
- Carrots, baby (1 pound)
- Cauliflower (1 head)
- Celery (6)
- Cilantro (1 bunch)
- Garlic (2 bulbs)
- Jicama (1)
- Lemons (2)
- Lime (1)
- Mushrooms, button (24 ounces)
- Onions, yellow (8)
- Orange juice (8 ounces)
- Parsley (1 bunch)
- Pears (4)
- Raspberries (2 pints)
- Rosemary (1 bunch)
- Salad greens (1 [10-ounce] bag)
- Spinach, baby (10 ounces)
- Strawberries (2 pints)
- Sweet potatoes (5)
- Swiss chard (1 bunch)
- Thyme (1 bunch)
- Zucchini (9 medium)

### DAIRY AND EGGS

- Eggs (3 dozen)
- Milk, almond (½ gallon)
- Yogurt, plain (24 ounces)

### MEAT

- Bacon, low-sodium, reduced-fat (12 ounces)
- Beef, ground, extra-lean (5 ounces)
- Chicken, drumsticks (4)
- Chicken, meaty bones (backs, wings) (4 pounds)
- Chicken, whole roaster (1)
- Cod (12 ounces)
- Fish, white (cod, halibut, snapper) (12 ounces)
- Pork, tenderloin (1 pound)
- Salmon (12 ounces)
- Turkey, breast (boneless, skinless) (12 ounces)
- Turkey, ground breast (1 pound)

### FROZEN

- Carrots, chopped (8 ounces)
- Mixed vegetables (1 pound)
- Peas (8 ounces)

### CANNED

- Applesauce, unsweetened (8 ounces)
- Black beans (1 [14-ounce] can)
- Capers (1 [2-ounce] jar)
- Coconut milk, lite (5 [14-ounce] cans)
- Pumpkin purée (1 [14-ounce] can)
- Tomatoes and green chiles, diced (such as Ro-Tel) (1 [14-ounce] can)
- Tomatoes, diced (1 [14-ounce] can)

### NUTS AND SEEDS

- Almonds (4 ounces)
- Pumpkin seeds, hulled (4 ounces)

## WEEK 4

### PRODUCE

- Apples (3)
- Apples, dried (½ cup)
- Banana (1)
- Blueberries (1 pint)
- Carrots (10)
- Celery (4)
- Garlic (2 bulbs)
- Jicama (1)
- Kale (2 bunches)
- Lemons (7)
- Lime (1)
- Mushrooms, button (1 pound)
- Onions, yellow (6)
- Orange juice (16 ounces)
- Peaches (2)
- Plums (2)
- Raspberries (2 pints)
- Spinach, baby (10 ounces)
- Squash, butternut (2)
- Squash, yellow (1 medium)
- Swiss chard (1 bunch)
- Zucchini (7 medium)

### DAIRY AND EGGS

- Eggs (3 dozen)
- Milk, almond (½ gallon)
- Yogurt, plain (24 ounces)

### MEAT

- Bacon, low-sodium, reduced-fat (8 ounces)
- Fish, white (cod, flounder) (12 ounces)
- Salmon (12 ounces)
- Shrimp, medium (12 ounces)
- Turkey, breast (boneless, skinless) (12 ounces)

### FROZEN

- Carrots, chopped (1 pound)
- Green beans (1 pound)

### CANNED

- Applesauce, unsweetened (8 ounces)
- Black beans (1 [14-ounce] can)
- Chiles, chopped green (1 [2-ounce] can)
- Coconut milk, lite (6 [14-ounce] cans)

### NUTS AND SEEDS

- Almonds (4 ounces)

# Conversion Tables

## Volume Equivalents (Liquid)

| US STANDARD | US STANDARD (OUNCES) | METRIC (APPROXIMATE) |
|---|---|---|
| 2 tablespoons | 1 fl. oz. | 30 mL |
| ¼ cup | 2 fl. oz. | 60 mL |
| ½ cup | 4 fl. oz. | 120 mL |
| 1 cup | 8 fl. oz. | 240 mL |
| 1½ cups | 12 fl. oz. | 355 mL |
| 2 cups or 1 pint | 16 fl. oz. | 475 mL |
| 4 cups or 1 quart | 32 fl. oz. | 1 L |
| 1 gallon | 128 fl. oz. | 4 L |

## Oven Temperatures

| FAHRENHEIT | CELSIUS (APPROXIMATE) |
|---|---|
| 250°F | 120°C |
| 300°F | 150°C |
| 325°F | 165°C |
| 350°F | 180°C |
| 375°F | 190°C |
| 400°F | 200°C |
| 425°F | 220°C |
| 450°F | 230°C |

## Volume Equivalents (Dry)

| US STANDARD | METRIC (APPROXIMATE) |
|---|---|
| ⅛ teaspoon | 0.5 mL |
| ¼ teaspoon | 1 mL |
| ½ teaspoon | 2 mL |
| ¾ teaspoon | 4 mL |
| 1 teaspoon | 5 mL |
| 1 tablespoon | 15 mL |
| ¼ cup | 59 mL |
| ⅓ cup | 79 mL |
| ½ cup | 118 mL |
| ⅔ cup | 156 mL |
| ¾ cup | 177 mL |
| 1 cup | 235 mL |
| 2 cups or 1 pint | 475 mL |
| 3 cups | 700 mL |
| 4 cups or 1 quart | 1 L |

## Weight Equivalents

| US STANDARD | METRIC (APPROXIMATE) |
|---|---|
| ½ ounce | 15 g |
| 1 ounce | 30 g |
| 2 ounces | 60 g |
| 4 ounces | 115 g |
| 8 ounces | 225 g |
| 12 ounces | 340 g |
| 16 ounces or 1 pound | 455 g |

# The Dirty Dozen and The Clean Fifteen

A nonprofit environmental watchdog organization called Environmental Working Group (EWG) looks at data supplied by the US Department of Agriculture (USDA) and the Food and Drug Administration (FDA) about pesticide residues. Each year it compiles a list of the best and worst pesticide loads found in commercial crops. You can use these lists to decide which fruits and vegetables to buy organic to minimize your exposure to pesticides and which produce is considered safe enough to buy conventionally. This does not mean they are pesticide-free, though, so wash these fruits and vegetables thoroughly.

These lists change every year, so make sure you look up the most recent one before you fill your shopping cart. You'll find the most recent lists, as well as a guide to pesticides in produce, at EWG.org/FoodNews.

## Dirty Dozen

| | |
|---|---|
| Apples | Strawberries |
| Celery | Sweet bell peppers |
| Cherries | Tomatoes |
| Cherry tomatoes | *In addition to the Dirty Dozen, the EWG added two types of produce contaminated with highly toxic organo-phosphate insecticides:* |
| Cucumbers | |
| Grapes | |
| Nectarines | |
| Peaches | |
| Spinach | Kale/Collard greens |
| | Hot peppers |

## Clean Fifteen

| | |
|---|---|
| Asparagus | Kiwis |
| Avocados | Mangoes |
| Cabbage | Onions |
| Cantaloupe | Papayas |
| Cauliflower | Pineapples |
| Eggplant | Sweet corn |
| Grapefruit | Sweet peas (frozen) |
| Honeydew melon | |

# Recipe Index

# Index

# About the Author

LAURA RELLIHAN is a registered dietitian, licensed nutritionist, and founder of her private nutrition practice, Back to Balance. Laura graduated from the University of Florida and completed her dietetic residency through the Bay Pines Veterans Health Care System.

Laura's strong interest in nutrition and a healthy lifestyle started at a young age, when she was diagnosed with systemic lupus erythematosus. After years of chemotherapy and other harsh medications, Laura realized that without good nutrition, her quality of life and health would not allow her to do the daily activities she enjoyed. Not only does Laura take pride in seeing her clients and families achieve their nutrition and health goals, but she also identifies with her clients' personal struggles because of her own health background.

In her free time, Laura enjoys being with her family, training and competing in triathlons, backpacking with her husband, and creating healthy recipes in her kitchen.